Prescribing in
Dermatology

The introduction of non-medical prescribing has meant that nurses, pharmacists and the professions allied to health are frequently faced with prescribing decisions. This text provides safe and effective information upon which to base these decisions when prescribing for patients with dermatological conditions. Each chapter looks at a common skin disorder (including acne vulgaris and rosacea, psoriasis, eczema, urticarias and angio-oedema, infections and infestations, and skin cancer) and provides information on assessment, differential diagnosis, management strategies and prescribing. Key background information from the relevant life sciences (anatomy, physiology, and pharmacology), as applied to clinical practice, is also provided. This book provides an invaluable guide for those healthcare professionals prescribing for, and treating, patients with dermatological conditions.

Prescribing in
Dermatology

Polly Buchanan

Molly Courtenay

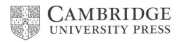

CAMBRIDGE
UNIVERSITY PRESS

CAMBRIDGE UNIVERSITY PRESS
Cambridge, New York, Melbourne, Madrid, Cape Town, Singapore, São Paulo

CAMBRIDGE UNIVERSITY PRESS
The Edinburgh Building, Cambridge CB2 2RU, UK

Published in the United States of America by Cambridge University Press, New York

www.cambridge.org
Information on this title: www.cambridge.org/9780521673785

First published 2006

Printed in the United Kingdom at the University Press, Cambridge

A catalogue record for this publication is available from the British Library

Library of Congress Cataloguing in Publication data

ISBN-13   978-0-521-67378-5   paperback
ISBN-10   0-521-67378-X   paperback

Every effort has been made in preparing this publication to provide accurate and up-to-date
information, which is in accord with accepted standards and practice at the time of publication.
Although case histories are drawn from actual cases, every effort has been made to disguise the
identities of the individuals involved. Nevertheless, the authors, editors and publishers can make
no warranties that the information contained herein is totally free from error, not least because
clinical standards are constantly changing through research and regulation. The authors, editors
and publishers therefore disclaim all liability for direct or consequential damages resulting from
the use of material contained in this publication. Readers are strongly advised to pay careful attention to information provided by the manufacturer of any drugs or equipment that they plan to use.

Contents

Preface

The introduction of non-medical prescribing has meant that nurses, pharmacists, and the professions allied to health are frequently faced with prescribing decisions. This text has been written for healthcare professionals involved in the treatment management of patients with dermatological conditions. Easily accessible information, upon which to base prescribing decisions ensuring safe and effective practice, is provided in the form of a single, easy to use, practice based text.

Each chapter looks at a common skin disorder. Information on assessment, differential diagnosis, and management is presented by Polly Buchanan. Background information from the relevant life sciences and key prescribing information is presented by Molly Courtenay. This book, in conjunction with the NPF/BNF, Drug Tariff and manufacturers' product information sheets, provides an essential guide for those healthcare professionals prescribing in the area of dermatology.

Polly Buchanan
Molly Courtenay
May 2006

Basic pharmacology

An appropriate knowledge and understanding of pharmacology is essential for those health care professionals prescribing in dermatology. It will influence decision-making with regards to the most appropriate medicine, the route of administration, the dose and frequency, potential contraindications, adverse effects and interactions with other drugs. This chapter provides fundamental information regarding pharmacokinetics and pharmacodynamics, and highlights issues that should be considered when assessing patients with respect to prescribing medication. A list of other useful textbooks has been provided at the end of the chapter, for those health care professionals wishing to read further.

Routes of administration

Drugs may act locally or systemically. Locally implies that the effects of the drug are confined to a specific area. Systemically means that the drug has to enter the vascular and lymphatic systems for delivery to body tissues. The main route of administration to provide a local effect is topical, whilst oral or parenteral administration of drugs are the main routes to provide a systemic effect. Some topical drugs can, however, have systemic effects, especially if given in large doses, in frequent doses or over a long period of time.

Topical administration

Topical preparations may be applied to the skin, mouth, nose, oropharynx, cornea, ear, urethra, vagina or rectum. These preparations may be administered in a variety of forms including:

- creams
- ointments
- gels
- lotions
- aerosols
- foams
- plasters
- powders
- patches
- suppositories
- sprays

Oral administration

This route of administration, which implies 'by mouth', is most commonly used. It tends to be convenient, simple and usually safe. Preparations may be in a solid form and include:

- tablets
- capsules
- powders
- granules
- lozenges

Other preparations may be provided in a liquid form and include:

- solutions
- emulsions
- suspensions
- syrups
- elixirs
- tinctures

Parenteral administration

Parenteral administration of a drug refers to the giving of a preparation by any route other than the gastrointestinal tract, by which a drug is injected or infused. This, therefore, includes intradermal, subcutaneous, intramuscular, intravenous, intrathecal and intra-articular routes. These sterile preparations are presented in ampules, vials, cartridges or large-volume containers.

Pharmacokinetics

Pharmacokinetics considers the movement of drugs within the body and the way in which the body affects drugs with time. Once a drug has been administered by one of the routes previously described, it will then undergo four basic processes:

1. Absorption
2. Distribution
3. Metabolism
4. Excretion

The composition of the drug has an important influence on where the drug is absorbed, where the drug is distributed to, where and how effectively it is metabolised and finally how rapidly it is excreted. In addition, other factors such as the dose of drug, the client's condition, and other therapeutic and environmental issues may also affect the effectiveness of these processes.

Each of these processes will now be considered in more detail.

Drug absorption

The process of absorption brings the drug from the site of administration into the circulatory or lymphatic system. Almost all drugs, other than those administered intravenously or some that are applied topically, must be absorbed before they can have an effect on the body. The term *bioavailability* is used to refer to the proportion of the administered drug that has reached the circulation, and that is available to have an effect. Drugs given intravenously may be considered to be 100% bioavailable as they are administered directly into the circulation and all of the drug may potentially cause an effect. Administration by other routes means that some of the drug molecules will be lost during absorption and distribution, and thus bioavailability is reduced.

Drugs administered orally are absorbed from the gastrointestinal tract, carried via the hepatic portal vein to the liver, and then undergo some metabolism by the liver before the drug has even had the opportunity to work. This removal of a drug by the liver, before the drug has become available for use, is called the *first-pass effect.* Some drugs, when swallowed and absorbed, will be almost totally inactivated by the first-pass effect (e.g. glyceryl trinitrate). The first-pass effect can, however, be avoided if the drug is given by another route. Thus, glyceryl trinitrate, when administered sublingually or transdermally, avoids first-pass metabolism by the liver and is able to cause a therapeutic effect.

Absorption following oral administration

For drugs given by all routes other than the intravenous route, several lipid cell membrane barriers will have to be passed before the drug reaches the circulation. Four major transport mechanisms exist to facilitate this process.

- *Passive diffusion* is the most important and the most common. If the drug is present in the gastrointestinal tract in a greater concentration that it is in the bloodstream, then a concentration gradient is said to exist. The presence of the concentration gradient will carry the drug through the cell membrane and into the circulation. The drug will be transported until the concentrations of drug are equal on either side of the cell membrane. No energy is expended during this process.
- *Facilitated diffusion* allows low-lipid-soluble drugs to be transported across the cell membrane by combining with a carrier molecule. This also requires a concentration gradient and expends no energy.
- *Active transport* is only used by drugs which closely resemble natural body substances. This process works against a concentration gradient, and requires a carrier molecule and energy to be expended.
- *Pinocytosis* or 'cell-drinking' is not a common method for absorbing drugs. It requires energy and involves the cell membrane invaginating and engulfing a fluid-filled vesicle or sac.

Factors affecting drug absorption from the gastrointestinal tract

A number of factors may influence the absorption of a drug from the gut. These include:

- *Gut motility*: If motility is increased and therefore transit time is reduced, there will be less time available for absorption of a drug. Hypomotility may increase the amount of drug absorbed if contact with the gut epithelium is prolonged.
- *Gastric emptying*: If increased, this will speed up drug absorption rate. If delayed, it will slow the delivery of drug to the intestine, therefore reducing the absorption rate.

- *Surface area*: The rate of drug absorption is greatest in the small intestine due to the large surface area provided by the villi.
- *Gut pH*: The pH of the gastrointestinal tract varies along its length. The changing environmental pH may have different effects on different drugs. Optimal absorption of a drug may be dependent on a specific pH.
- *Blood flow*: The small intestine has a very good blood supply which is one reason why most absorption occurs in this part of the gut. Faster absorption rates will occur in areas where blood supply is ample.
- *Presence of food and fluid in the gastrointestinal tract*: The presence of food in the gut may selectively increase or decrease drug absorption. For example, food increases the absorption of dicoumarol, whilst tetracycline absorption is reduced by the presence of dairy foods. Fluid taken with medication will aid dissolution of the drug and enhance its passage to the small intestine.
- *Antacids*: The presence of these in the gastrointestinal tract causes a change in environmental pH. They will increase absorption of basic drugs and decrease absorption of acidic ones.
- *Drug composition*: Various factors pertaining to the composition of the drug may affect the rate at which it is absorbed. For example, liquid preparations are more rapidly absorbed than solid ones, the presence of an enteric coating may slow absorption, and lipid-soluble drugs are rapidly absorbed.

Absorption following parenteral administration

Intradermal drugs diffuse slowly from the injection site into local capillaries, and the process is a little faster with drugs administered subcutaneously. Due to the rich supply of blood to muscles, absorption following an intramuscular injection is even quicker. The degree of tissue perfusion and condition of the injection site will influence the rate of drug absorption.

Absorption following topical administration

Drugs applied topically to the mucous membranes and skin are absorbed less than by oral and parenteral routes. Absorption is, however, increased if the skin is broken or if the area is covered with an occlusive dressing.

Rectal and sublingual absorption is usually rapid due to the vascularity of the mucosa. Absorption from instillation into the nose may lead to systemic as well as local effects, whilst inhalation into the lungs provides for extensive absorption. Minimal absorption will occur from instillation into the ears, but absorption from the eyes depends on whether a solution or ointment is administered.

Drug distribution

This process involves the transportation of the drug to the target site of action. During distribution, some drug molecules may be deposited at storage sites and others may be deposited and inactivated. Various factors may influence how and even if, a drug is distributed.

- *Blood flow*: Distribution may depend on tissue perfusion. Organs that are highly vascular such as the heart, liver and kidneys will rapidly acquire a drug. Levels of a drug in bone, fat, muscle and skin may take some time to rise due to reduced vascularity. The client's level of activity and local tissue temperature may also affect drug distribution to the skin and muscle.
- *Plasma protein binding*: In the circulation, a drug is bound to circulating plasma proteins or is 'free' in an un-bound state. The plasma protein usually involved in binding a drug is albumin. If a drug is bound, then it is said to be inactive and cannot have a pharmacological effect. Only the free drug molecules can cause an effect. As free molecules leave the circulation, drug molecules are released from plasma protein to re-establish a ratio between the bound and the free molecules. Binding tends to be non-specific and competitive. This means that plasma proteins will bind with many different drugs and these drugs will compete for binding sites on the plasma proteins. Displacement of one drug by another drug may have serious consequences. For example, warfarin can be displaced by tolbutamide producing a risk of haemorrhage, whilst tolbutamide can be displaced by salicylates producing a risk of hypoglycaemia.
- *Placental barrier*: The chorionic villi enclose the foetal capillaries. These are separated from the maternal capillaries by a layer of trophoblastic cells. This barrier will permit the passage of lipid-soluble, non-ionised compounds from mother to foetus but prevents entrance of those substances that are poorly lipid-soluble.
- *Blood–brain barrier*: Capillaries of the central nervous system differ from those in most other parts of the body. They lack channels between endothelial cells through which substances in the blood normally gain access to the extracellular fluid. This barrier constrains the passage of substances from the blood to the brain and cerebrospinal fluid. Lipid-soluble drugs

(e.g. diazepam), will pass fairly readily into the central nervous system, where as lipid-insoluble drugs will have little or no effect.

- *Storage sites*: Fat tissue will act as a storage site for lipid-soluble drugs (e.g. anticoagulants). Drugs that have accumulated there, may remain for some time, not being released until after administration of the drugs has ceased. Calcium-containing structures such as bone and teeth can accumulate drugs that are bound to calcium (e.g. tetracycline).

Drug metabolism

Drug metabolism or *biotransformation* refers to the process of modifying or altering the chemical composition of the drug. The pharmacological activity of the drug is usually removed. Metabolites (products of metabolism) are produced which are more polar and less lipid-soluble than the original drug, which ultimately promotes their excretion from the body. Most drug metabolism occurs in the liver, where hepatic enzymes catalyze various biochemical reactions. Metabolism of drugs may also occur in the kidneys, intestinal mucosa, lungs, plasma and placenta.

Metabolism proceeds in two phases:

- *Phase I*: These reactions attempt to biotransform the drug to a more polar metabolite. The most common reactions are oxidations, catalysed by mixed function oxidase enzymes. Other Phase I reactions include reduction and hydrolysis reactions.
- *Phase II*: Drugs or Phase I metabolites which are not sufficiently polar for excretion by the kidneys, are made more hydrophilic ('water-liking') by conjugation (synthetic) reactions with endogenous compounds provided by the liver. The resulting conjugates are then readily excreted by the kidneys.

With some drugs, if given repeatedly, metabolism of the drugs becomes more effective due to enzyme induction. Therefore larger and larger doses of the drug become required in order to produce the same effect. This is referred to as *drug tolerance*.

Tolerance may also develop as a result of adaptive changes at cell receptors. Various factors affect a client's ability to metabolise drugs. These include:

- *Genetic differences*: The enzyme systems which control drug metabolism are genetically determined. Some individuals show exaggerated and prolonged responses to drugs such as propranolol which undergo extensive hepatic metabolism.

- *Age*: In the elderly, first-pass metabolism may be reduced, resulting in increased bioavailability. In addition, the delayed production and elimination of active metabolites may prolong drug action. Reduced doses may, therefore, be necessary in the elderly. The enzyme systems responsible for conjugation are not fully effective in the neonate and this group of clients may be at an increased risk of toxic effects of drugs.
- *Disease processes*: Liver disease (acute or chronic) will affect metabolism if there is destruction of hepatocytes. Reduced hepatic blood flow as a result of cardiac failure or shock may also reduce the rate of metabolism of drugs.

Drug excretion

Kidneys

Most drugs and metabolites are excreted by the kidneys. Small drug or metabolite molecules may be transported by glomerular filtration into the tubule. This, however, only applies to free drugs and not drugs bound to plasma proteins. Active secretion of some drugs into the lumen of the nephron will also occur. This process however, requires membrane carriers and energy.

Several factors may affect the rate at which a drug is excreted by the kidneys. These include:

- Presence of kidney disease (e.g. renal failure).
- Altered renal blood flow.
- pH of urine.
- Concentration of the drug in plasma.
- Molecular weight of the drug.

Bile

Several drugs and metabolites are secreted by the liver into bile. These then enter the duodenum via the common bile duct, and move through the small intestine. Some drugs will be reabsorbed back into the bloodstream and return to the liver by the enterohepatic circulation (Figure 1.1). The drug then undergoes further metabolism or is secreted back into bile. This is referred to as enterohepatic cycling and may extend the duration of action of a drug. Drugs secreted into bile, will ultimately pass through the large intestine and be excreted in faeces.

Lungs

Anaesthetic gases and small amounts of alcohol undergo pulmonary excretion.

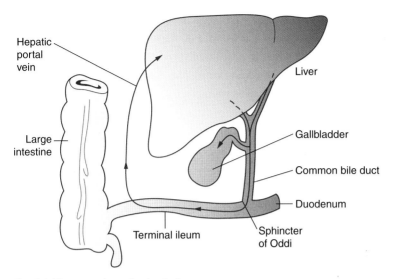

Fig. 1.1 The enterohepatic circulation.

Breast milk

Milk-producing glands are surrounded by a network of capillaries, and drugs may pass from maternal blood into the breast milk. The amounts of drug may be very small, but may affect a suckling infant who has less ability to metabolise and excrete drugs.

Perspiration, saliva and tears

Drugs may be excreted passively via these body secretions if the drugs are lipid-soluble.

The processes of drug metabolism and drug excretion will ultimately determine the drug's *half-life*. This is the time taken for the concentration of drug in the blood to fall by half (50%) its original value. Standard dosage intervals are based on half-life calculations. This helps in the setting up of a dosage regime which produces stable plasma drug concentrations, keeping the level of drug below toxic levels but above the minimum effective level.

There are occasions when an effective plasma level of drug must be reached quickly. This requires a dose of the drug which is larger than is normally given. This is called a *loading dose*. Once the required plasma level of drug has been reached, the normal recommended dose is given. This is then continued at regular intervals to maintain a stable plasma level and is called the *maintenance dose*.

Determining plasma levels of a drug at frequent intervals is undertaken when clients are prescribed drugs with a narrow *therapeutic index* (e.g. digoxin and lithium). The therapeutic index is the ratio of the drug's toxic dose to its minimally effective dose. Monitoring plasma levels can also be used to assess a client's compliance to drug therapy.

Pharmacodynamics

Whilst pharmacokinetics considers the way in which the body affects a drug by the processes of absorption, distribution, metabolism and excretion, pharmacodynamics considers the effects of the drug on the body and the mode of drug action.

All body functions are mediated by control systems which depend on enzymes, receptors on cell surfaces, carrier molecules and specific macromolecules (e.g. DNA). Most drugs act by interfering with these control systems at a molecular level. In order to have their effect, drugs must reach cells via the processes of absorption and distribution already described. Once at their site of action, drugs may work in a very specific manner or non-specifically. Specific mechanisms will be considered first of all.

- *Interaction with receptors on the cell membrane*: A receptor is usually a protein molecule found on the surface of the cell or located intracellularly in the cytoplasm. Drugs frequently interact with receptors to form a drug-receptor complex. In order for a drug to interact with a receptor, it has to have a complementary structure in the same way that a key has a structure complementary to the lock in which it fits (Figure 1.2). Very few drugs are truly specific to a particular receptor and some drugs will combine with

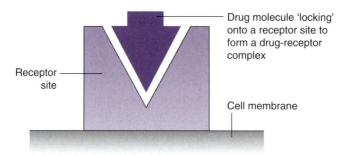

Fig. 1.2 Drug-receptor complex.

more than one type of receptor. However, many drugs show selective activity on one particular receptor type.

A drug that has an affinity for a receptor, and that once bound to the receptor can cause a specific response, is called an *agonist*. Morphine is an opioid agonist that binds to mu receptors in the central nervous system to depress the appreciation of pain. Drugs that bind to receptors and do not cause a response are called *antagonists* or receptor blockers. These will reduce the likelihood of another drug or chemical binding and hence will reduce or block further drug activity. Antagonists may be *competitive*, in which case they compete with an agonist for receptor sites and inhibit the action of the agonist. The action of the drug depends on whether it is the agonist or antagonist which occupies the most receptors. For example, naloxone is a competitive antagonist for mu receptors and is may be used to treat opioid overdose. It will compete with morphine for mu receptors and reverse the effects of an excessive dose of morphine. A *non-competitive* antagonist will inactivate a receptor so that an agonist cannot have an effect.

Drug-receptor binding is reversible and the response to the drug is gradually reduced once the drug leaves the receptor site.

- *Interference with ion passage through the cell membrane*: Ion channels are selective pores in the cell membrane that allow the movement of ions in and out of the cell. Some drugs will block these channels, which ultimately interferes with ion transport and causes an altered physiological response. Drugs working in this way include nifedipine, verapamil and lignocaine.
- *Enzyme inhibition or stimulation*: Enzymes are proteins and biological catalysts which speed up the rate of chemical reactions. Some drugs interact with enzymes in a manner similar to the drug-receptor complex mechanism already described. Drugs often resemble a natural substrate and compete with the natural substrate for the enzyme. Drugs interacting with enzymes include aspirin, methotrexate and angiotensin-converting enzyme (ACE) inhibitors such as enalapril.
- *Incorporation into macromolecules*: Some drugs may be taken up by a larger molecule and will interfere with the normal function of that molecule. For example, when the anticancer drug 5-fluorouracil is incorporated into messenger RNA, taking the place of the molecule uracil, transcription is affected.
- *Interference with metabolic processes of micro-organisms*: Some drugs interfere with metabolic processes that are very specific or unique to micro-organisms and thus kill or inhibit activity of the micro-organism. Penicillin

disrupts bacterial cell wall formation whilst trimethoprim inhibits bacterial folic acid synthesis.

Non-specific mechanisms involve:

- *Chemical alteration of the cellular environment*: Drugs may not alter specific cell function, but because they alter the chemical environment around the cell, cellular responses or changes occur. Drugs which have this effect include osmotic diuretics (e.g. mannitol), osmotic laxatives (e.g. lactulose) and antacids (e.g. magnesium hydroxide).
- *Physical alteration of the cellular environment*: Drugs may not alter specific cell function, but because they alter the physical as opposed to the chemical environment around the cell, cellular responses or changes occur. Drugs which have this effect would include docusate sodium which lowers faecal surface tension and many of the barrier preparations available, which protect the skin.

Undesirable responses to drug therapy

Most drugs are not entirely free of unwanted effects. However, drugs which are frequently prescribed, highly potent or that have a narrow therapeutic index, are likely to increase the risk of unwanted effects.

Terms used to describe undesirable responses to drugs include:

- *Adverse reaction*: This refers to any undesirable drug effect.
- *Side effect*: This is used interchangeably with the term adverse reaction. It refers to unwanted but predictable responses to a drug.
- *Toxic effect*: This usually occurs when too much drug has accumulated in the client. It may be due to an acute high dose of a drug, chronic buildup over time or increased sensitivity to the standard dose of a drug.
- *Drug allergy (hypersensitivity)*: The body sees the drug as an antigen and an immune response is established against the drug. This may be an immediate response or delayed.

Factors affecting an individual's response to a drug

Many individual factors will determine an individual's clinical response to a drug. Some of these have already been identified but additional factors will also be considered here. The prescriber should be fully aware of these factors and they should be incorporated into the client assessment before decisions are made about which drug to prescribe. In addition, they should be considered when monitoring drugs which are already being used by the client, whether the drugs are prescribed or obtained 'over-the-counter'.

- *Age*: The very young and the elderly particularly have problems related to their ability to metabolise and excrete drugs. Neonatal hepatic enzyme systems are not fully effective, so drug metabolism will be reduced and there is an increased risk of toxicity. In the elderly, delayed metabolism by the liver and a decline in renal function means delayed excretion by the kidneys and drug action may be prolonged. Complicated drug regimes may be difficult for the elderly to follow which may mean inadequate or excessive doses of drugs are consumed.
- *Body weight*: The size of an individual will affect the amount of a drug that is distributed and available to act. The larger the individual, the larger the area for drug distribution. Lipid-soluble drugs may be sequestered in fat stores and not available for use. This is the reason that some drugs are given according to the client's body weight (i.e. x milligrams per kilogram of body weight). All clients should have their weight recorded and this should be reassessed regularly if the client is receiving long-term drug treatment.
- *Pregnancy and lactation*: Lipid-soluble, unionised drugs in the free state will cross the placenta (e.g. opiates, warfarin). Some may be teratogenic and cause foetal malformation. Drugs can also be transferred to the suckling infant via breast milk and have adverse effects on the child (e.g. sedatives, anticonvulsants and caffeine). A full drug history should be obtained pre-conception where possible or as soon as pregnancy has been diagnosed. Women must be educated not to take medication without consulting a physician, pharmacist, midwife or nurse.
- *Nutritional status*: Clients who are malnourished may have altered drug distribution and metabolism. Inadequate dietary protein may affect enzyme activity and slow the metabolism of drugs. A reduction in plasma protein levels may mean that more free drug is available for activity. A loss of body fat stores will mean less sequestering of the drug in fat and more drug available for activity. Normal doses in the severely malnourished may lead to toxicity. Nutritional assessment of clients is, therefore, essential and malnutrition should be managed accordingly.
- *Food-drug interactions*: The presence of food may enhance or inhibit the absorption of a drug. For example, orange juice (vitamin C) will enhance

the absorption of iron sulphate, but dairy produce reduces the absorption of tetracycline. Monoamine oxidase inhibitors must not be taken with foods rich in tyramine, such as cheese, meat yeast extracts, some types of alcoholic drinks and other products, due to toxic effects occurring, such as a sudden hypertensive crisis. Nurses should have some knowledge of common food-drug interactions and drug administration may need timing in relation to mealtimes.

- *Disease processes*: Altered functioning of many body systems will affect an individuals response to a drug. Only a few examples are therefore given.
  - Changes in gut motility and therefore transit time may affect absorption rates (e.g. with diarrhoea and vomiting absorption is reduced). Loss of absorptive surface in the small intestine, as occurs in Crohn's disease will affect absorption.
  - Hepatic disease (e.g. hepatitis, cirrhosis and liver failure) will reduce metabolism of drugs and lead to a gradual accumulation of drugs and risk of toxicity.
  - Renal disease (e.g. acute and chronic renal failure) will reduce excretion of drugs and drugs may accumulate.
  - Circulatory diseases (e.g. heart failure and peripheral vascular disease) will reduce distribution and transport of drugs.
- *Mental and emotional factors*: Many factors may affect a client's ability to comply with their drug regime. These include confusion, amnesia, identified mental illness, stress, bereavement and many others. These types of problems may lead to inadequate or excessive use of medication resulting in unsuccessful treatment or serious adverse effects. The nurse must consider these issues in the client assessment.
- *Genetic and ethnic factors*: Enzyme systems controlling drug metabolism are genetically determined and therefore, genetic variation leads to differences in clients' abilities to metabolise drugs. For example, some individuals possess an atypical form of the enzyme pseudocholinesterase. When these individuals are given the muscle relaxant suxamethonium, prolonged paralysis occurs and recovery from the drug takes longer.

Different races of people are also known to dispose of drugs at different rates.

FURTHER READING

Baer CL & Williams BR (1996) *Clinical Pharmacology and Nursing*, 3rd edn. Springhouse, PA: Springhouse Corporation.

Clarke JB, Queener SF & Karb V (1997) *Pharmacologic Basis of Nursing Practice*, 5th edn. St Louis: Mosby.

Downie G, Mackenzie J & Williams A (2003) *Pharmacology and Medicines Management for Nurses*, 3rd edn. Edinburgh: Churchill Livingstone.

Galbraith A, Bullock S, Manias E, Richards A & Hunt B (1999) *Fundamentals of Pharmacology: A Text for Nurses and Health Professionals.* Singapore: Addison Wesley Longman.

McGavock H (2003) How drugs work. Oxford: Radcliffe Medical Press.

Pinnell NL (1996) *Nursing Pharmacology.* Philadelphia: W.B. Saunders.

Rang HP, Dale MM & Ritter JM (1999) *Pharmacology*, 4th edn. Edinburgh: Churchill Livingstone.

Springhouse (2001) *Clinical Pharmacology Made Incredibly Easy!* Springhouse, PA: Springhouse Corporation.

Trounce JR & Gould D (2000) *Clinical Pharmacology for Nurses*, 16th edn. Edinburgh: Churchill Livingstone.

2

The skin

This chapter provides a brief description of the anatomy and physiology of the skin. This will aid understanding of the various conditions that affect the skin, together with the recommended treatment management.

The skin is the largest of the body's organs. It has a vast surface area, which spans approximately $2\,m^2$ and accounts for roughly 16% of an individual's total body weight. The skin (see Figure 2.1) is composed of two major layers of tissue: the outer epidermis and the inner dermis. It also has a number of accessory structures including hair, nails, sweat glands and sebaceous glands. These structures, although located in the dermis, protrude through the epidermis to the skin surface.

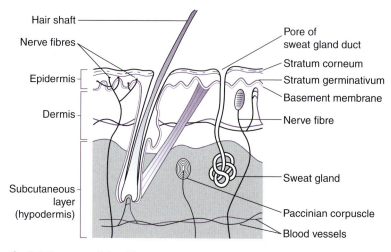

Fig. 2.1 Structure of the skin.

The skin has a number of functions (Martini 2000). These include:

- Protection of underlying organs and tissues.
- Excretion of waste products, salts and water.
- Maintenance of normal body temperature.
- Storage of nutrients.
- Detection of stimuli such as temperature, and the relay of this information to the nervous system.

The epidermis

The skin is persistently subjected to mechanical injury. The epidermis provides protection, and also prevents micro-organisms from entering the body. It is comprised of a number of layers. The innermost layer of the epidermis is called the stratum germinativum, and the outermost layer, the stratum corneum. The stratum germinativum is attached to a basement membrane which separates the dermis from the epidermis.

The stratum germinativum is composed of many germinative or basal cells, the division of which replace the cells shed at the epithelial surface. As these germinative cells move towards the skins surface, their structure and activity changes. Whilst still at the basal layer, they begin forming a protein called keratin. The formation of this protein is continued as they move towards the skin's surface. Eventually, as the cells reach the stratum corneum, approximately 15–30 days later, they are like flattened bags of protein, and their intracellular organelles have disappeared.

Before they are lost from the stratum corneum, these cells remain in this layer for a further 2 weeks. This provides the underlying tissue with a protective barrier of cells, which although dead, are exceedingly durable. The stratum corneum is the major barrier to the loss of water from the body. It has two actions, which restrain the movement of water and limit the loss of water from the skin's surface. Firstly, the matrix in which the cells of the stratum corneum are embedded is rich in lipid. This substance is almost impenetrable to water and therefore makes it extremely difficult for water molecules to move out of the epidermal cell. Secondly, protein inside the epidermal cells attracts, and holds on to water molecules. As a consequence of these actions, the surface of the skin is therefore normally dry, with very little water lost and so is, therefore, unsuitable for the growth of many micro-organisms. Although water-resistant, the stratum corneum is not waterproof. Interstitial fluid gradually penetrates this layer of tissue to be evaporated from the surface into the surrounding air. Approximately 500 ml is lost from the body each day in this way.

Dermis

The dermis is comprised of a network of two types of protein. These proteins are collagen and elastin. The collagen fibres provide strength to the skin. The elastin gives the skin its flexibility. The dermis is also comprised of a network of blood vessels, and a number of other structures. These include:

(a) *Sweat glands*: Millions of these glands are found in the dermis all over the body. Eccrine sweat glands are more common and are found mainly in the palms, soles and forehead. When the temperature of the body rises due to emotional stress, a hot environment or exercise, eccrine glands become activated. Evaporation of these secretions on the skins surface causes cooling. Apocrine sweat glands are found in the mammary, anal, genital and axillary surfaces of the body. These glands become active during sexual arousal and emotional stress.

(b) *Sebaceous glands*: These glands produce sebum and are found all over the body (except the palms of the hands or soles of the feet) and in close proximity to body hair. Sebum is an oil comprising fatty acids, substances toxic to bacteria and cholesterol. Sebum is secreted into the hair follicle by means of the sebaceous duct. The skin and the hair are kept soft by movement of the sebum along the hair shaft to the skins surface.

(c) *Nails*: Nails are keratinised epidermal cells which protect the fingers and toes.

(d) *Hair*: The hair base or bulb, is situated in the dermis. The papilla is a pointed projection of the dermis protruding into the hair bulb. The cells of the hair follicle (which house the hair root found beneath the skin) are nourished by the papilla. The cells near the surface of the hair follicle are hard and keratinised.

There are variations in the structure of the skin in relation to age, environment and ethnic origin. The skin also varies between different parts of the body. For example, non-hairy (glabrous) skin (e.g. on the palms of hands and soles of feet) has an extremely thick epidermis and numerous sensory receptors.

The skin with hair follicles, hairy skin (e.g. on the scalp) has a thin epidermis and many sebaceous glands.

REFERENCE

Martini FH (2000) *Fundamentals of Anatomy and Physiology*, 5th edn. New Jersey: Prentice Hall International.

3

Treatment of infection

This chapter deals with the different groups of antibacterials that are available to treat established infections. The structure of a generalised bacterial cell is provided in Figure 3.1.

Surrounding the bacterial cell, is a cell wall containing peptidoglycan. This substance is unique to bacteria and not found in human cells. Within the cell wall is the selectively permeable bacterial cell membrane. This is similar to the human cell, in that it consists of a phospholipid bilayer and membrane proteins, but it does not contain sterols. The cytoplasm is found within the cell membrane. As in human cells, the cytoplasm contains soluble proteins (many enzymes), ribosomes for protein synthesis, inorganic ions and intermediary molecules of metabolism. The bacterial cell, unlike the human cell, has no nucleus. The genetic material exists in a single chromosome lying within the cytoplasm.

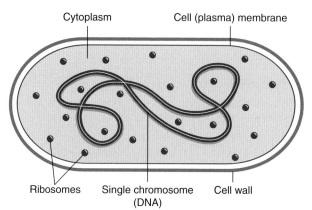

Cytoplasm   Cell (plasma) membrane

Ribosomes   Single chromosome   Cell wall
              (DNA)

Fig. 3.1 Structure of a bacterial cell.

Antibacterial drugs can be classified in several ways:

1. They can be described as being bacteriostatic or bacteriocidal. Bacteriostatic drugs inhibit bacterial growth without killing the cell. The human immune system will ultimately destroy the organism. Bacteriocidal drugs kill the bacteria.
2. By chemical structure.
3. According to their mode of action (described later in this chapter).
4. According to their range or spectrum of activity. They may be 'broad spectrum' or 'narrow spectrum'.

Groups of antibacterial drugs

Antibacterial drugs can be classified into groups according to their chemical structure. Examples of these groups include:

- Penicillinase-resistant penicillins, e.g. Flucloxacillin.
- Broad-spectrum penicillins, e.g. Amoxycillin.
- Tetracyclines, e.g. Tetracycline, doxycycline, minocycline, oxytetracycline, lymecycline.
- Aminoglycosides, e.g. Tetracycline, doxycycline, minocycline, oxytetracycline, lymecycline.
- Aminoglycosides, e.g. Gentamycin, neomycin.
- Macrolides, e.g. Erythromycin.

Other antibacterials include chloramphenicol, fusidic acid, trimethoprim, metronidazole, nitrofurantoin, clindamycin.

Mode of action

There are five major mechanisms by which antibacterial drugs have their effect (Wingard *et al.* 1991). These are:

- Inhibition of synthesis and damage to the bacterial cell wall.
- Inhibition of synthesis and damage to the bacterial cell membrane.
- Modification of bacterial nucleic acid synthesis.
- Inhibition or modification of bacterial protein synthesis.
- Modification of bacterial energy metabolism.

Inhibition of synthesis and damage to the bacterial cell wall

Penicillins, penicillinase-resistant penicillins, broad spectrum penicillins and cephalosporins all disrupt formation of the peptidoglycan layer of the cell wall. The bacterial cell is then unable to maintain its osmotic gradient and begins to swell. Eventually the cell ruptures and dies.

Inhibition of synthesis and damage to the bacterial cell membrane

Polymyxins bind to membrane phospholipids and alter permeability to sodium and potassium ions. Holes are generated in the membrane and this disrupts the cell's osmotic gradient. The cell eventually ruptures.

Modification of bacterial nucleic acid synthesis

Quinolones inhibit replication of bacterial deoxyribonucleic acid (DNA). They block the activity of DNA gyrase, an enzyme essential for DNA replication and repair. Metronidazole acts via an intermediate which inhibits the synthesis of bacterial DNA and breaks down existing DNA. The precise action of nitrofurantoin is not established. It is thought that the drug is reduced to an unstable metabolite which causes DNA strand breakage and bacterial damage.

Inhibition or modification of bacterial protein synthesis

Several groups of antibacterials prevent the production of essential bacterial cell proteins. Tetracyclines, aminoglycosides, macrolides, clindamycin and chloramphenicol all act by binding to one of the subunits of the bacterial ribosomes where proteins are actually manufactured, and hence prevent protein synthesis. Fusidic acid prevents transfer ribonucleic acid (tRNA) binding to the ribosomes. Protein synthesis inhibitors tend to have bacteriostatic properties.

Modification of bacterial energy metabolism

Trimethoprim acts by inhibition of the folate pathway in bacteria. Bacteria have to synthesise their own folate derivatives which are important in intracellular reactions. Trimethoprim interrupts the conversion of dihydrofolic acid to tetrahydrofolic acid, by inhibiting the enzyme dihydrofolate reductase.

Contraindications

- *Penicillins*: Penicillin hypersensitivity.
- *Tetracyclines*: Renal impairment, pregnancy and breast feeding, children under 12 years.
- *Aminoglycosides*: Myasthenia gravis, hypersensitivity.
- *Macrolides*: Hypersensitivity. Estolate contraindicated in hepatic disease.
- *Chloramphenicol*: Pregnancy and breast feeding, porphyria.
- *Fusidic acid*: Hypersensitivity.
- *Trimethoprim*: Renal impairment and blood dyscrasias.
- *Metronidazole*: Hypersensitivity.
- *Nitrofurantoin*: G6PD deficiency, impaired renal function and in infants under 3 months old.
- *Clindamycin*: Diarrhoeal states.

Side-effects

- Penicillins and penicillinase-resistant penicillins

Oral preparations of phenoxymethylpenicillin and flucloxacillin may cause: hypersensitivity reactions (urticaria, fever, joint pains, rashes, angioedema, anaphylaxis), haemolytic anaemia, interstitial nephritis, thrombocytopenia, neutropenia, paraesthesia, diarrhoea and antibiotic-associated colitis.

- Broad spectrum penicillins

Oral preparations of amoxycillin and co-amoxiclav may cause: nausea, vomiting, diarrhoea, rashes, hypersensitivity reactions (urticaria, fever, joint pains, rashes, angioedema, anaphylaxis), haemolytic anaemia, interstitial nephritis, thrombocytopenia, neutropenia and paraesthesia.

- Tetracyclines

Oral preparations of tetracycline, doxycycline, minocycline, lymecycline and oxytetracycline may cause: nausea, vomiting, diarrhoea, dysphagia, oesophageal irritation, hypersensitivity (rash, urticaria, angioedema, anaphylaxis, exfoliative dermatitis), headache, visual disturbance, hepatotoxicity, pancreatitis, photosensitivity, blood dyscrasias and skin discolouration.

- Aminoglycosides

Gentamycin and neomycin are included in topical preparations and may cause irritation, burning, stinging and itching.

- Macrolides

Oral preparations of erythromycin and clarithromycin may cause: nausea, vomiting, abdominal discomfort, diarrhoea, urticaria, rashes and other allergic reactions, reversible hearing loss, cholestatic jaundice and cardiac effects. Clarithromycin may in addition cause dyspepsia, headache, smell and taste disturbance, stomatitis, glossitis, myalgia, arthralgia, dizziness, vertigo, tinnitus, anxiety, insomnia, nightmares, confusion, psychosis, jaundice and hepatitis.

Topical erythromycin may cause mild irritation of the skin and sensitisation.

- Chloramphenicol

Topical chloramphenicol may cause transient stinging.

- Fusidic acid

Rarely, hypersensitivity to topical administration has been reported.

- Trimethoprim

Oral trimethoprim may cause: nausea, vomiting, rashes, pruritus, hyperkalaemia and depression of haematopoiesis, photosensitivity and allergic reactions (angioedema and anaphylaxis).

- Metronidazole

Oral metronidazole may cause: nausea, vomiting, rashes, furred tongue, drowsiness, headache, dizziness, ataxia, urticaria, pruritus, angioedema, anaphylaxis, hepatitis, jaundice, myalgia, joint pains, thrombocytopenia and aplastic anaemia.

Vaginal application of metronidazole gel may cause: local irritation, abnormal discharge, candidiasis and increased pelvic pressure.

- Nitrofurantoin

Oral nitrofurantoin may cause: nausea, vomiting, anorexia, diarrhoea, peripheral neuropathy, acute and chronic pulmonary reactions, angioedema, urticaria, rash, pruritus, jaundice, hepatitis, pancreatitis, arthralgia and blood dyscrasias.

- Clindamycin

Topical clindamycin may cause mild irritation of the skin and sensitisation. Clindamycin vaginal cream may damage latex condoms and diaphragms.

Before prescribing an antibacterial, the following factors should be considered:

1. Previous history of antibacterial therapy, previous history of allergy, present hepatic and renal function, and other previously listed contra-indications.
2. The dose of drug to be prescribed will depend on several factors including age, weight and renal function.
3. Local antibacterial policies may indicate which drugs should be prescribed and these documents should be consulted by the prescriber.
4. Viral infections should not be treated with antibacterials.
5. Antibacterials should not be prescribed prophylactically.
6. Specimens should be obtained from the affected site for culture and sensitivity so the causative organism can be identified. When the organism has been isolated, treatment may be changed to another drug if deemed more appropriate.
7. Some oral antibacterials should be administered at specific times:
   - Amoxycillin and phenoxymethylpenicillin are not affected by gastric acid and can be taken without concern about meals.
   - Tetracycline should be administered on an empty stomach. It should be taken 1 hour before meals or 2 hours after. Calcium, aluminium, iron, Magnesium, bismuths, zinc salts, quinopril, antidiarrhoeals, antacids and dairy products will adversely affect absorption of tetracyclines. Absorption of lymecycline, doxycycline and minocycline is not significantly impaired by moderate amounts of milk. Doxycycline and minocycline can be taken on a full or empty stomach (Galbraith *et al.* 1999). All tetracyclines should be swallowed whole while sitting or standing.
   - Nitrofurantoin should be taken after meals to avoid gastric irritation.

The patient should receive education about timing and spacing of medication, side-effects and the importance of completing the prescribed course. If allergic reactions occur, the drug should be discontinued and a physician notified immediately.

REFERENCES

Galbraith A, Bullock S, Manias E, Richards A & Hunt B (1999) *Fundamentals of Pharmacology: A Text for Nurses and Health Professionals.* Singapore: Addison Wesley Longman.

Wingard LB, Brody TM, Larner J & Schwartz A (1991) *Human Pharmacology: Molecular to Clinical.* St Louis: Mosby Year Book.

4

Acne vulgaris and rosacea

Acne vulgaris and rosacea are chronic inflammatory skin conditions which characteristically flare during acute episodes. Both conditions are associated with the development of facial erythema, papules and pustules. Differential diagnosis is important as treatment varies depending on the stage and severity of each condition. The psychological impact of acne vulgaris or rosacea can be profound therefore early intervention is always advocated. Table 4.1 denotes the main clinical differences between acne and rosacea.

Acne vulgaris

Acne vulgaris (see Figures 4.1 and 4.2) represents one of the most common skin conditions seen in primary care (Layton 1999). Acne involves the pilosebacious

Table 4.1 Main clinical differences between acne vulgaris and rosacea.

Acne	Rosacea
• underlying seborrhoea	• no seborrhoea
• presence of comedones	• no comedones
• more common in teenagers	• more common in middle ages
• more common in males	• more common in females
• affects face, chest and back	• more common in fair skinned persons
• less facial erythema	• usually only the face is affected
• presence of scarring	• presence of telangiectasia (dilated superficial blood vessels)

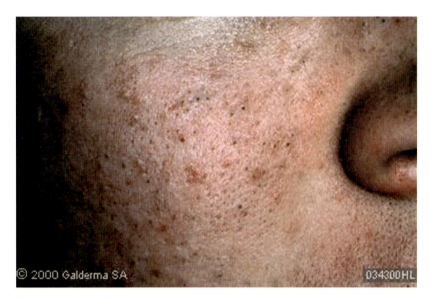

Fig. 4.1 Acne comedones.

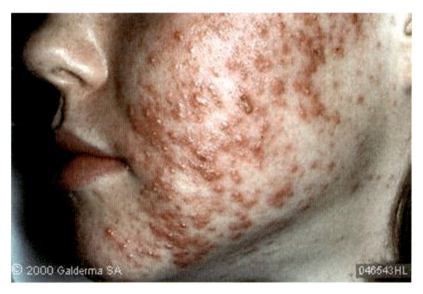

Fig. 4.2 Acne inflamed.

units (PSUs) of the skin. PSUs consist of a sebaceous gland connected to a canal, called a follicle, that contains a fine hair (see Figure 4.3). These units are most numerous on the face, upper back and chest, and acne predominantly affects these areas.

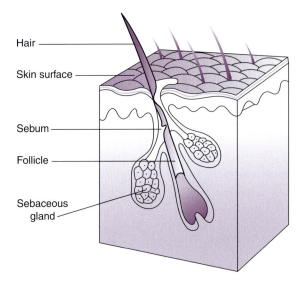

Fig. 4.3 A PSU.

The onset of acne vulgaris is frequently occurs in early adolescence and can persist for many years (age range 11–30). Occasionally, acne can appear in early childhood or infancy (juvenile acne) or persist into the fourth decade of life (Cunliffe & Gould 1979). An understanding of the pathogenesis of acne is vital in the successful management of this condition.

Four distinct patho-physiological factors contribute to the development and severity of acne.

1. Increased sebum production. An increase in androgens during puberty causes the sebaceous glands to enlarge and produce greater amounts of sebum. This causes the skin to become greasy (seborrhoea).
2. Blockage of the follicular duct. The cells lining the follicular duct act abnormally to testosterone. They become sticky and are not shed normally. This causes a blockage of the follicular duct and prevents the flow of sebum from the sebaceous gland. Sebum collects in the duct and this gives rise to blackheads and whiteheads (comedones).
3. Colonisation of *Propionibacterium acnes* bacteria within follicular ducts and the production of inflammatory chemicals.
4. Penetration of the dermis with inflammatory chemicals causing the skin to become red and swollen with the development of pustules (raised lesions containing white or yellow purulent fluid).

Table 4.2 Acne severity and clinical appearance.	
Severity of acne	Clinical appearance
Mild	Seborrhoea; Predominantly comedonal lesions; Presence of open and closed comedones (blackheads and whiteheads respectively); Micro-comedones (the first stage of comedo formation, a comedo so small that it can be seen only with a microscope present); papular lesions (inflamed lesions) $+/-$ inflammation
Moderate	Seborrhoea; open and closed comedones papular and pustular lesion with inflammation
Severe	Seborrhoea; open and closed comedones; papular and pustular inflammatory lesions; scarring; $+/-$ nodulo-cystic lesions (deep-nodular lesions with or without inflammatory component sometimes called an acne 'cyst').

All managements should be targeted towards resolving the four contributing factors of acne vulgaris. This involves consideration of the distribution and severity of seborrhoea, comedones, inflammatory lesions, pustular lesions and nodulo-cystic lesions and scarring.

Assessment

An accurate patient assessment is paramount in the management of patients with acne vulgaris. As well as taking a general history, the physiological *and psychological* needs of the patient must be assessed. Acne requires mid to long-term management (months–years) with topical or/and systemic therapies. The success of any therapy is dependent on patient concordance and this requires ongoing support and advice from prescribers. Prescribers have an important role in accurately assessing the clinical, psychological and educational needs of individual patients. The following sections outlines a clear assessment strategy to assist prescribers make clinical decisions regarding the most appropriate therapies for patient presenting with acne.

General history
- *Past medical history*: Past medical illnesses and operations, presence of polycystic ovarian syndrome, previous skin disease (especially in childhood),

history of allergy or sensitivities, prescribed medications, over-the-counter medications, herbal remedies and vitamins.

- *Family history*: Acne, rosacea, seborrhoea, autoimmune diseases, allergies, familial diseases, presence of polycystic ovarian syndrome.
- *Social history*: Occupation, leisure and sport interests, home situation, travel abroad, pets and animals.

Physiological assessment

- Clinical history of skin lesions and acne development:
  - Duration of acne: How and when did lesions begin to appear?
  - What types of lesions are present (open/closed comedones, papules, pustules, cystic lesions, scarring)?
  - Site of acne.
  - Does anything make your acne better or worse?
  - Is your acne painful?
  - Do you pick or squeeze your spots?
- Presence and description of lesion(s):
  - Comedones (closed and open) appear as whiteheads and blackheads, respectively.
  - Papules (raised lesion <5 mm) appear as inflamed lesions.
  - Pustules (raised lesions containing white or yellow purulent fluid).
  - Cystic lesions (deep nodular lesions with or without inflammatory component).
  - Scarring lesions often described as 'ice-pick' in appearance.
  - Hypo/hyper-pigmentation of skin or lesions (post-inflammatory hyper-pigmentation).
  - Hypertrophic scars and keloid scarring (especially in darker skin types).
- Distribution of lesions:
  - The presence of comedones confirms the diagnosis of acne vulgaris.
  - Lesions are usually polymorphic, multiple, localised or widespread.
  - Typically, acne affects the seborrhoeic areas of the skin (e.g. face, chest and back).

Clinical assessment

- Morphology of lesions:
  - Comedones and microcomedones are the precursor lesions of acne vulgaris.
  - Closed comedones appear as small-firm papules or 'whiteheads'.

- Open comedones appear as small-firm papules or 'blackheads' (due to oxidisation of surface sebum).
- Inflammatory papular lesions appear due to accumulation of *P. acnes* bacterium in blocked PSU initiating an inflammatory reaction.
- Pustules appear due to the accumulation of debris during and following the inflammatory process.
- Cystic lesions are deeper lesions within the dermis.
- Scarring occurs following healing or resolution of inflammatory dermal lesions.

Psychological assessment

Psychological morbidity such as anxiety and depression is frequently reported in patients with acne. Acne sufferers can develop a low self-esteem, which can impact on all aspects of the persons personal, social and working relationships.

- Psychological impact:

Self concept: From the patient's perspective, How does the skin appears to others? How does the patient (and others) react to this?

Self image: How does the patient cope with the look of his/her skin?

Concordance: How has the patient coped with current/previous treatments?

- What is the patient's understanding in relation to the disease, treatment and prognosis and are there any knowledge deficits?
- Patient's willingness in being involved in decisions about their skin treatments, previous satisfaction or dissatisfaction with treatments or progress.
- What are the patient's expectations of the treatment prescribed?

Layton (2004) supports the use of the Assessment of Psychological and Social Effects of Acne (APSEA) scale which was developed in Leeds and can be used with a generic Quality of life scale and or patient satisfaction tool.

If using a clinical and/or psychological assessment tool, it is important to document serial measurements to assess progress and satisfaction. They can help reassure the patient that progress is being made or help reassure the health professional that referral to a specialist is appropriate.

General daily skin care

Daily cleansing of the skin is important as part of the management programme. Excessive washing and cleansing is not necessary and will further irritate inflamed and delicate skin. Use of a mild soap or soap substitute to gently wash the affected skin helps to reduce seborrhoea. Some commercially available products claim to be anticomedonal which can help reduce comedone development. Use of abrasive substances in washes and cleansers have to be used with caution. Excessive use can irritate and damage delicate skin causing inflammation and abrasions. Generally oil free moisturising products and makeups are advocated for persons with acne.

Patients should be advised to control the desire to pick and squeeze the lesions as this can further traumatise the skin, and induce further inflammation and scarring. Early management of comedones and micro-comedones help reduce the development of inflammatory lesions. Therefore maintenance therapy, using anti-comedonal agents (e.g. topical retinoids), during non-inflammatory phases should be considered.

Preparations for the treatment of acne vulgaris

Preparations used to treat acne include:

1. Benzoyl peroxide and azelaic acid
2. Retinoids
3. Antimicrobials: Antibiotics

Benzoyl peroxide and azelaic acid

Mode of action Benzoyl peroxide unblocks sebaceous glands by removing the top layer of skin (keratolytic effect). Inflammation of the blocked follicle is reduced as this preparation also kills the bacteria causing the infection. Benzoyl peroxide can also be used in combination with an antimicrobial agent. These products have both a keratolytic and antimicrobial action. Azelaic acid has a similar action to benzoyl peroxide.

Caution Benzoyl peroxide should not be allowed to come into contact with the mouth, mucous membranes or eyes. It can cause bleaching of fabrics and hair and patients should avoid excessive exposure to sunlight.

Side effects Benzoyl peroxide and azelaic acid can cause skin irritation particularly when therapy is commenced. This usually subsides if treatment is continued at a reduced frequency or, if treatment is suspended until irritation subsides and re-introduced at a reduced frequency.

It is reasonable to expect a 50% improvement in skin condition for patients using topical treatments at 3 month review. If no improvement is demonstrated within 3 months, alternative therapy should be considered and can include alternative monotherapies or adding in another topical therapy (combination).

Retinoids

Mode of action Retinoids reduce sebum production and enable the drainage of sebum by causing the epidermal layer to be less cohesive. Topical retinoids include:

- Adapalene
- Tretinoin
- Isotretinoin

Contraindications Retinoids should not be applied during pregnancy or, if breast feeding. Tretinoin is contraindicated if an individual has a history of cutaneous epithelioma.

Cautions These preparations should not be applied when acne covers a large surface area. Contact with eyes, nostrils, mouth, mucous membranes and broken skin should be avoided. Exposure to ultraviolet light and cosmetic astringents should also be avoided.

Side effects The side effects of retinoids include local burning, erythema, stinging, pruritus, dry or peeling skin. During the initial stages of treatment with tretinoin, acne can become exacerbated.

Isotretinoin can be prescribed orally for acne. This drug is teratogenic and should not be given to pregnant women or women who are likely to become pregnant and not practising effective contraception. It is also contraindicated during breastfeeding or in individuals with renal of hepatic impairment. This drug has many side effects commonly including chelitis, dermatitis, nose bleeds and headaches. More severe side effects include hyperlipidaemia, hepatotoxicity and neutropaenia.

Antimicrobials (Antibiotics)

Topical preparations of erythromycin, tetracycline or clindamycin are effective in the treatment of acne. Antibacterial resistance of *P. acnes* is increasing.

Therefore where possible:

- Use non-antibiotic antimicrobials (e.g. benzoyl peroxide or azelaic acid).
- Avoid concomitant with different oral and topical antibiotics.
- Use an effective antibiotic for a repeat course if needed (3–6 months).

- Inform patients that the skin may take 2–3 months to show an improvement.
- Don't continue treatment for longer than necessary (British National Formulary (BNF) 2005). Regular 3 monthly follow-up is advised.

Oral antibiotics may be prescribed if topical treatment is not effective. Preparations include oxytetracycline, tetracycline, lymecycline, doxycycline and minocycline (see Chapter 3 for mode of action, contraindications and side effects of these preparations). Lymecycline demonstrates less epigastric problems associated with the tetracycline antibiotics. Furthermore, lymecycline is a once a day preparation and this may improve adherence to treatment regime.

Hormone treatment

Co-cyprindiol which contains an anti-androgen can be used to treat acne. It is useful in women who also wish to receive oral contraception.

Willingness and suitability of this mode of treatment should be discussed as part of the assessment strategy and patients advised accordingly to consult with their general practitioner (GP).

Summary action of main acne treatments   The main groups of drugs used in the management of acne are specifically targeted towards:

Benzoyl peroxide	Comedones and inflamed lesions.
Topical retinoids	Anti-comedonal and anti-inflammatory. Treats precursor lesions (comedones) which helps prevent progression to inflammatory lesions. Important in both active and maintenance therapies.
Topical antimicrobials	Anti-inflammatory and anti-comedonal. Helps reduce colonisation of *P. acnes* bacterium and subsequent inflammatory response.
Topical/systemic antibiotics	Reduces colonisation of *P. acnes* and inflammatory response.
Systemic retinoids	Anti-inflammatory, anti-comedonal and help reduce hypercornification of follicular ducts.
Systemic antiandrogens	Reduces sebum production and sebaceous gland hyperplasia.

Table 4.3 Acne treatment algorithm (Gollnick *et al.* 2003).

	Mild		Moderate		Severe
	Comedonal acne	Papular/pustular acne	Papular/pustular acne	Nodular acne (nodules >0.5–1 cm)	Nodular/conglobate acne
First choice	topical retinoid	topical retinoid + topical antimicrobial	Oral antibiotic + topical retinoid +/– benzoyl peroxide	Oral antibiotic + topical retinoid +/– benzoyl peroxide	Oral isotretinoin (2nd course incase of relapse)
Alternative choice	Alternative topical retinoid OR azelaic acid OR salicylic acid	Alternative topical antimicrobial agent + alternative topical retinoid OR azelaic acid	Alternative oral antibiotic + alternative topical retinoid +/– benzoyl peroxide	Oral isotretinoin OR alternative oral antibiotic + alternative topical retinoid +/– benzoyl peroxide	High-dose oral antibiotic + topical retinoid + benzoyl peroxide
Alternatives for *females*	See first choice	See first choice	Oral antiandrogen + topical retinoid/azelaic acid +/– benzoyl peroxide	Oral antiandrogen + topical retinoid +/– oral antibiotic +/– alternative antimicrobial	High-dose oral antiandrogen + topical retinoid +/– alternative topical antimicrobial
Maintenance therapy	Topical retinoid	Topical retinoid +/– benzoyl peroxide			

The Leeds Revised Acne Grading System (Gollnick *et al.* 2003) (see Table 4.3) is an algorithm to assess the clinical severity of acne and can be useful in clinical decisions regarding appropriate treatment regimens.

Rosacea

Rosacea is a chronic inflammatory skin condition of unknown aetiology (see Figure 4.4). It occurs in persons whose skin is prone to flushing therefore it has been postulated that the underlying defect is vascular in nature. Rosacea affects 1–10% of the population, it is more predominant in the middle aged and females. Paler skin types, such as celts, northern European and the fair skinned are more

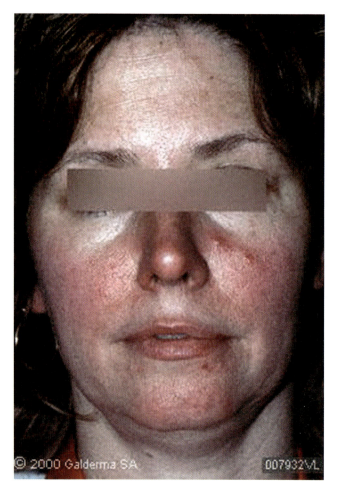

Fig. 4.4 Acne rosacea.

prone to developing rosacea (Plewig & Kligman 2000). It is characterised by the development of a erythematous rash on the cheeks. The nose, forehead, scalp and eyes can become affected. The facial redness becomes persistent often with the presence of dilated blood vessels over cheeks. Acute episodes of papules, pustules and oedema can occur in response to various triggers. These episodes can persist for weeks (British Association of Dermatologists (BAD) 2005).

Three distinct stages are recognised in the development of rosacea:

- Stage 1
  - Persistent facial erythema
  - Telangiectasia on cheeks, nose, forehead
  - Sensitive, irritable skin
  - Stinging and burning sensation on application of cosmetics and treatment creams
- Stage 2
  - Development of papules, pustules and lymphoedema
  - Skin follicles affected and sebaceous glands enlarged
  - Prominent facial pores
  - Extension of rash over face and scalp
- Stage 3
  - Persistent oedematous, inflamed facial skin
  - Facial contours become thickened, coarse and irregular
  - Tissue overgrowth especially nose, chin, eyelids, ears and forehead
  - Ocular involvement with inflammation, irritation, erythema, discomfort, photosensitivity
  - Ocular keratitis with impaired vision

Triggers to acute flares

Certain substances and conditions are thought to trigger acute episodes of rosacea:

- Foods triggers
  - Coffee, tea, chocolate, cold drinks, alcohol, soy sauce, cheese, citrus fruits, curries, vinegar, tomatoes, red meat, yogurt
  - Large meals
  - Thermal heat
  - Highly spiced foods, pickled foods, smoked foods, fermented foods
- Chemical triggers
  - Caffeine, vasodilators, perfumes, aftershaves, astringents, cosmetics

- Environmental triggers
  - Resident Demodex skin mite in follicles and sebaceous glands
  - Gastrointestinal upset (e.g. diarrhoea, cholecystitis, gastritis)
  - Weather conditions (e.g. Sunlight, wind)
  - Heat and cold
- Other triggers
  - Topical corticosteroids

Assessment

As with acne, both physiological and psychological assessment is important in the successful management of rosacea.

This includes:

- Onset, duration and distribution of rash
- Past medical history/previous episodes of rosacea
- Family history
- Description and type of lesions
- Severity of condition/erythema, telangiectasia, oedema, contour changes, discomfort
- Previous medication for rosacea
- Concomitant medications
- Occupational and social history
- Triggers to acute flares
- Psychological assessment
  - Embarrassment, anxiety, depression
  - Disruption of lifestyle

General skin care advice

- Avoid or reduce exposure to known triggers
- Protect skin from sunshine (application of sunblock Sun Protection Factor (SPF) 15+)
- Gentle washing and cleansing of facial skin will reduce irritation
- Use non irritating soap substitutes, cleansers, makeups
- Wash off shampoos away from the facial area
- Cosmetic camouflage can help reduce obvious erythema
- Seek medical advice early if rosacea becomes severe or affects the eyes

Treatment

Rosacea can be managed by topical and systemic medications (vann Zuuren *et al.* 2003). Complete resolution is unlikely with treatment, however early intervention can effectively reduce and control the severity of underlying erythema and acute flares. More severe cases may also require tertiary referral for specialist treatments for example, laser therapy for telangiectasia, or plastic surgery for rhinophyma (bulbous nose).

Topical therapies for rosacea

- Metronidazole cream or gel (see Chapter 3)
- Azelaic acid cream (see section Acne vulgaris)
- Daily sunblock SPF 15+

Use of topical corticosteroids is contraindicated for rosacea as they cause increased erythema, telangiectasia and pustule formation.

Topical acne preparations such as retinoids, and benzoyl peroxide can irritate the skin and are not advised in the management of rosacea.

Systemic therapies for rosacea

- Long-term tetracycline antibiotics (10–12 weeks) (see Chapter 3)
- Erythromycin antibiotics considered if no response to tetracyclines
- Antidepressants if evidence of depression
- Beta-blockers for facial flush if severe
- Isotretinoin considered in very severe cases under specialist supervision (see section Acne vulgaris)

Specialist referral

Three key groups of patients with acne or rosacea warrant specialist referral (Chu 2004):

1. Appropriate referrals
   (a) Patients who have failed to respond to conventional therapy and who are at risk of scarring.
   (b) Patients who require medications or treatments prescribed by specialists (e.g. laser therapy, dermabrasion, peels, systemic isotretinoin).
   (c) patients with profound psychological morbidity (e.g. anxiety, depression).

(d) Patients with rosacea and ocular involvement should be referred to an eye specialist.

2. Delayed referrals

   (a) Patients who have delayed in seeking medical help early in the disease course.

   (b) Patients who have been referred too late for specialist help. Patients referred within 3 years of disease onset fair better, both clinically and psychologically.

3. Referrals after *inadequate* previous therapies

   (a) Oral antibiotics as monotherapy.

   (b) Oral antibiotics for less than 3–6 months.

   (c) Oral antibiotics for 12–24 months with no clinical improvement due to poor concordance.

   (d) Long-term (>6 months) topical monotherapies (e.g. antimicrobials, antibacterials).

   (e) Poor concordance due to knowledge deficit and lack of support.

REFERENCES

British Association of Dermatologists (BAD) (2005) *Patient Information Leaflet: Rosacea.* London: BAD. www.bad.org.uk/public/leflets/rosacea.asp

British National Formulary (BNF) (2005). British Medical Association (BMA). Royal Pharmaceutical Society of Great Britain (RPSGB). London: BMA and RPSGB.

Chu T (2004) When to refer to a dermatologist. In: *Acne: A Review of Current Treatments and Best Practice* (Ed. Cunliffe W). Round Table Series 80. London: The Royal Society of Medicine Press, 32–5.

Cunliffe W & Gould DJ (1979) Prevalence of facial acne vulgaris in late adolescence and in adults. *Br Med J* 1: 1109–10.

Gollnick H, Cunliffe WJ, Berson D *et al.* (2003) Management of acne: a report from a Global Alliance to improve outcomes in acne. *J Am Acad Dermatol* 49: s1–s37.

Layton A (1999) Acne – What's new? *Dermatol Pract*: 16–18.[AQ1]

Layton A (2004) Disease severity and assessment of acne. In: *Acne: A Review of Current Treatments and Best Practice* (Ed. Cunliffe). Round Table Series 80. London: The Royal Society of Medicine Press, pp. 5–9.

Plewig G & Kligman AM (2000) *Acne and Rosacea,* 3rd edn. New York: Springer-Verlag.

Van Zuuren EJ, Graber MA, Hollis S, Chaudhry M, & Gupta AK (2003) Interventions for rosacea. *The Cochrane Database of Systematic Reviews.* Issue 4. Art. No.: CD003262. DOI: 10.1002/14651858.CD003262.pub2.

5

Psoriasis

Psoriasis is a chronic inflammatory skin condition which affect approximately 3% of the population (Koo 1996). Psoriasis is a genetically determined condition (Elder *et al.* 2001) and occurs frequently in one or two generations of the same family (Leder *et al.* 1998).

Psoriasis involves the dermis and the epidermis of the skin and can appear anywhere on the body as raised erythematous scaly plaques, i.e. red, scaly patches of skin (see Figures 5.1–5.4). Psoriasis frequently occurs in adulthood and can persist for many years, with periods of relapse and remission. The extensor surfaces of the body (i.e. knees and elbows), scalp and natal cleft (between the buttocks) are particularly common sites of psoriasis. The nails may also be involved and this presents as pitting of the nail plate (i.e. the presence of small depressions on the nail surface) with more severe involvement causing onycholysis (i.e. loosening or separation of a nail from its bed) and nail destruction.

Although psoriasis is a genetically determined condition, certain predisposing factors or 'triggers to relapse' have been identified. These include:

1. trauma (physical, emotional and chemical)
2. hormones
3. medication
4. infection
5. sunlight.

The clinical sub-types of psoriasis are given in Table 5.1.

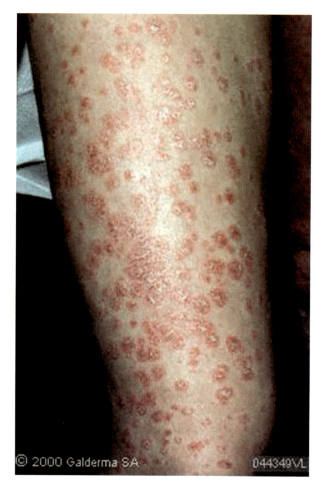

Fig. 5.1 Psoriasis
guttate.

Patho-physiological changes in the skin

The patho-physiological changes which occur as a result of psoriasis can be grouped into those which affect the epidermis and those which affect the dermis. Changes which affect the epidermis include:

- increased cell proliferation with hyperkeratosis, i.e. build up of skin scale on top of the epidermis;
- parakeratosis (white areas of the nail plate);
- acanthosis (thickening) of the epidermis – over-production of immature keratinocytes (squamous cells) which results in the typical white adherent mica scale associated with plaques.

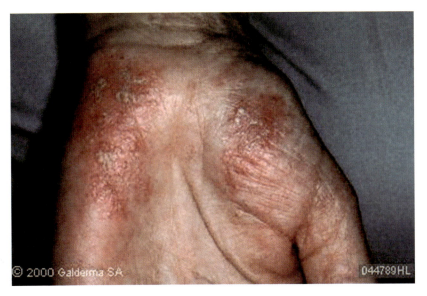

Fig. 5.2 Psoriasis (hand).

Dermal changes include:

- increased vascularisation;
- engorgement of the dermal blood vessels;
- mononuclear cell infiltration (infiltration of mononucleocytes from blood stream out with blood vessels, around skin appendages and in upper layer of dermis) which results in the characteristic erythematous plaques.

A further form of psoriasis (psoriatic arthropathy) is associated with inflammatory arthritis of the distal joints of the feet and hand.

Assessment

As well as taking a general history, the physiological and psychological needs of the patient must be assessed. Psoriasis requires long-term management (many years) with topical (or/and systemic therapies). The success of any therapy is dependent on patient concordance and this requires ongoing support and advice from prescribing health professionals. Prescribers have an important role in accurately assessing the clinical, psychological and educational needs of individual patients. The following sections outlines a clear assessment strategy to assist prescribers make clinical decisions regarding the most appropriate therapies for patient presenting with psoriasis.

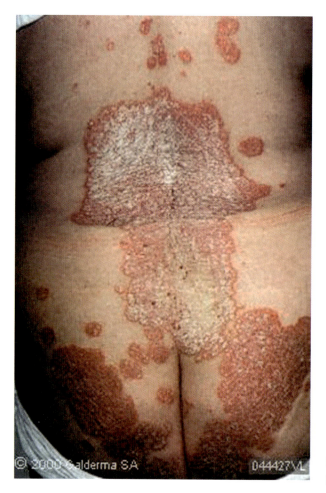

Fig. 5.3 Psoriasis plaque.

General history

- *Past medical history*: Age of patient. Age at onset of psoriasis. Past medical illnesses and operations, previous skin disease (especially in childhood or triggered by infection), history of allergy or sensitivities, prescribed medications, over-the-counter medications, herbal remedies and vitamins. Child bearing potential, desire to impregnate, liver disease, hypertension, smoking and alcohol intake (Higgins 2000).

- *Family history*: Psoriasis, eczema, autoimmune diseases, allergies, familial diseases.

- *Social history*: Occupation, leisure and sport interests, home situation, travel abroad, pets and animals. Potential trigger factors such as drugs, environment,

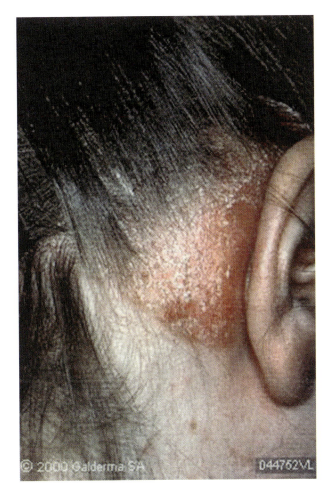

Fig. 5.4 Psoriasis.

stress, physical, chemical or emotional trauma. Coincidental-related disease, e.g. HIV. The ability to access treatment (community-based and hospital-based services).

Physiological assessment

- Clinical history of skin lesions and psoriasis development:
  - Duration of psoriasis: How and when did lesions begin to appear?
  - What types of lesions are present (plaques, scaling lesions, inverse lesions eyrthematous lesions, pustular lesions)?
  - Site of psoriasis lesions?
  - Does anything make your psoriasis better or worse?

Table 5.1 Clinical sub-types of psoriasis.

Type of psoriasis	Clinical appearance
Plaque (large and small)	Raised, erythematous plaques, hyperkeratosis (thickening of the outer layer of the skin) with mica scaling (fine powdery scale) and pruritus. Often extensor surfaces involved as well as lesions on trunk, scalp and limbs. Often excludes face.
Guttate	Extensive, small droplet like erythematous scaling lesions. Often triggered by streptococcal infection of the throat. Frequently affects young adults (Rasmussen 2000).
Scalp	Restricted to scalp. Erythematous scaling lesions can extend over entire scalp to hairline. Severe hyperkeratosis and scaling. Associated with amiantacea of scalp, that is a condition of the scalp characterised by thick, yellow-white scales densely coating the scalp skin and adhering to the scalp hairs as they exit the scalp.
Nail	Pitting, onycholysis, erythema and scaling of nail folds. Severe cases nail destruction.
Flexural (inverse)	Erythematous non-scaly lesions of flexures and intertrigenous areas (i.e. areas where two skin surfaces touch, e.g. under breasts, groin, finger and toe webs). Primary fungal infection can have a similar appearance in the sites. Secondary fungal infection on psoriatic lesions can occur in these sites and require antifungal treatments.
Localised palmar–plantar pustulosis	Erythematous, pustular lesions of palms of hands and soles of feet. Can involve nails.
Generalised pustular psoriasis	Unstable widespread form. Regarded as a dermatology emergency. Extensive erythematous pustular lesions over the entire body.
Erythrodermic psoriasis	Major dermatological emergency. General malaise. Unstable, frequently exfoliative (massive scaling of the skin) form. >95% skin erythematous. Loss of skin function i.e. temperature control, fluid control. Susceptible to infection. Requires urgent hospital admission.

- Is your psoriasis itchy or painful?
- Is there any joint involvement?
- Presence and description of lesions:
  - Plaque psoriasis (80–90% of patients): Small or large plaques of erthematous skin covered in fine silvery scale?
  - Guttate psoriasis: Papules (raised lesion <5 mm) appear as inflamed lesions.
  - Pustular psoriasis: Pustules (raised lesions containing white or yellow fluid).
  - Localised or generalised?
  - Annular lesions: Plaque psoriasis resolving from centre of lesion.
  - Hypo/hyper-pigmentation of skin or lesions (post-inflammatory residual hyperpigmentation, staining of skin due to treatment therapies, e.g. dithranol).
  - Pitting of nails?
  - Onycholysis of nails?
  - Erythodermic psoriasis?
  - Palmar–plantar psoriasis?
  - Scalp psoriasis?
  - Flexural (inverse) psoriasis, frequently smooth non-scaling lesions?
- Distribution of lesions:
  - Lesions can localised (elbows, knees, sacral region, scalp, palms and soles, flexures) or widespread over entire body including face, ears and genitalia.
  - Severity and extent of lesions: This involves estimating body surface area (BSA) affected and degree of erythema, induration (thickness of plaque) scaling, and itch or pain (see Psoriasis Area and Severity Index (PASI) score as cited in Mason *et al.* 2004).

Psychological assessment
Quality of life considerations are important. These will include ability to perform activities of daily living, employability, interpersonal relationships. Psychological morbidity such as anxiety and depression is frequently reported in patients with psoriasis. Psoriasis sufferers can develop a low self esteem, which can impact on all aspects of the person's personal, social and working relationships.

- Psychological impact
  - *Self Concept* (from the patient's perspective):
    - How does the skin appears to others?
    - How does the patient (and others) react to this?

   – *Self Image*:
      – How does the patient cope with the look of his/her skin?
   – *Concordance*:
      – How has the patient coped with current/previous treatments?
      – What is the patient's understanding in relation to the disease, treat-
        ment, and prognosis and are there any knowledge deficits? Patient's
        willingness in being involved in decisions about their skin treatments,
        previous satisfaction or dissatisfaction with treatments or progress.

If using a clinical and/or psychological assessment tool it is important to
document serial measurements to assess progress and satisfaction. These
tools can help reassure the patient that progress is being made, and also help
reassure the health professional that referral to a specialist is appropriate.

   It is important to include information from both the physiological and psychological assessments before categorising the severity of the psoriasis (i.e. mild,
moderate or severe). 'Mild' localised psoriasis may still warrant secondary care
referral if the patient's quality of life, activities and functioning has been affected.
However, as a general rule of thumb, mild to moderate psoriasis is managed on
an outpatient or home management basis using topical therapies. Moderate to
severe disease includes those patients with more than 5% BSA or those requiring
more aggressive therapies such those who have lesions on the hands, soles, scalp
and genitalia. Patient with psoriatic arthopathy may require more aggressive systemic treatments despite mild to moderate skin involvement.

   The management of all types of psoriasis should be targeted towards resolving the increased epidermal cell turnover and/or dermal inflammatory
response. This involves consideration of the distribution and severity of lesions.

Preparation for the treatment of psoriasis

The main groups of drugs used in the management of psoriasis are:

1. Emollients
2. Keratolytics
3. Topical tar
4. Topical dithranol
5. Vitamin D and its analogues
6. Retinoids
7. Topical corticosteroids
8. Systemic immunomodulators.

Emollients

Emollients soothe, smooth and hydrate the skin. These preparations help in psoriasis by reducing build up of keratinocytes and scale. They are particularly useful in inflammatory psoriasis and palmo-plantar plaque psoriasis. The effects of emollient preparations are short lived, and they need to be applied frequently even after improvement occurs. Emollient preparations are available in a variety of presentations. Each of these preparations varies with regard to the water and oil content of the mixture. Preparations with a high water content produce a greater cooling effect on the skin, and so are very effective for individuals suffering from pruritus. Individuals with very severe dry skin may benefit from an emollient with higher oil content. The high oil content produces a greater sealing effect on the skin, and thus prevents water evaporation to a greater extent.

Mode of action

Creams Creams are oil-in-water emulsions. Their action takes place in two stages (Nathan 1997). Firstly, following the initial application of the preparation, water is lost from the mixture by both evaporation, and absorption into the skin. This water evaporation has the effect of cooling the skin and alleviating pruritus. Secondly, the water loss from the mixture, combined with the mechanical stress of applying the preparation, causes the emulsion to crack. This cracking releases the oil phase. During this phase, oil is released onto the surface of the skin, sealing it and preventing any further water evaporating from the skin's surface.

Creams are generally well absorbed into the skin, are less greasy than ointments, and easier to apply. They therefore tend to be more cosmetically acceptable. Aqueous cream is an example of a cream preparation.

Ointments Ointments are greasy preparations, that do not normally contain water, and are insoluble in water. They are more occlusive than creams. Ointments are particularly effective in chronic, dry lesions. Commonly used ointment bases consist of soft paraffin or a combination of soft, liquid and hard paraffin. Emulsifying ointment is an example of this type of preparation.

A wide range of emollient preparations are currently available. However, there is little published evidence of the relative effectiveness of these products, and choice is often a matter of personal preference. All emollient products can be bought over the counter. However, some of these products may be very expensive, and are usually supplied on prescription.

The administration of an emollient will depend on the condition of the skin. It may be necessary for an individual to have a daily bath containing an emollient, and then to apply further emollients. In other instances, individuals may only require the infrequent application of cream to an area of dry skin. Individuals with severe dry skin will benefit from having a bath prior to using an emollient. The bath water will hydrate the skin and therefore provide an extremely good base for the application of these preparations. The bath water must only be lukewarm (approximately 37°(C)). This is very important, as if it is any hotter, blood vessels will become dilated and any itching may become worse. Emulsifying ointment can also be used as a bath additive. Approximately 30 gm of this mixture should be mixed with hot water and poured into the bath. Following bathing, the skin should be gently patted dry. If an emollient preparation is to be applied to the skin, it should be done so before the skin dries out, and immediately following the bath. Emollients can be applied as often as they are required throughout the day.

Contraindications

Generally, emollients are very safe to use, the only contraindication being sensitivity to the constituents in the preparation.

Enhanced emollients

Enhanced emollients contain substances which specifically promote or enhance the therapeutic effect. Common constituents of enhanced emollients are salicylic acid (keratolytic) which act as a de-scaling agent within the emollient. Natural moisturising factors (NMFs) are also commonly used to enhance the effect of otherwise simple emollients, such as Urea and Lactic acid. These NMFs aid penetration into dry skin and have an antimicrobial, anti-inflammatory effects. Enhanced emollients are particularly useful for very dry hyperkeratotic skin (Callen *et al.* 2003).

Topical tar

Mode of action

Coal tar is an anti-inflammatory and reduces scaling in psoriasis. Crude coal tar is smelly, stains and is difficult to apply. Concordance is therefore a common problem. Refined tar preparations are available and more cosmetically acceptable. Tar preparations include shampoos, bath emollients, scalp applications, creams, lotions and ointments.

Caution

Avoid eyes, mucosa, genital or rectal areas, and broken or inflamed skin (BNF 2005).

Contraindications

Do not use in sore, acute or pustular psoriasis or in the presence of an infection (BNF 2005).

Side effects

Skin irritation and acne-like eruptions, photosensitivity. Stains skin, hair and fabric (BNF 2005).

Topical dithranol

Mode of action

Dithranol is more potent than coal tar and requires expert management. It is very effective in chronic plaque psoriasis. It is commonly used in secondary care as an intensive therapy, as a 24 hour application (in lassar's paste), or as a short contact therapy (30 minute application). It can also be used in conjunction with Ultraviolet Light Therapy as Modified Inghram's Regime (Storbeck *et al.* 1993, Ingram 1953). Dithranol acts by diminishing cellular proliferation. Proprietary short contact preparations are available for home use but careful support and education is required.

Cautions

Dithranol can cause severe skin irritation. It must only be applied to the affected area and surrounding skin must be protected. Gloves must be worn when this preparation is applied and any contact (especially with the eyes) must be avoided.

Contraindications

Hypersensitivity, acute and pustular psoriasis (BNF 2005).

Side effects

Local burning sensation and irritation. When applied, the skin is stained purple/brown. Furniture and clothing can also become stained. Although skin staining fades within 2/3 weeks, this makes home management difficult.

Vitamin D3 and derivatives

Mode of action

Calcipotriol, calcitriol and tacalcitol are analogues of vitamin D3. Calcitriol is the naturally occurring active form of vitamin D3. All vitamin D3 derivatives inhibit cell proliferation and stimulate differentiation of keratinocytes thereby normalising cell turnover characterised in psoriasis. Vitamin D3 derivatives are indicated for mild to moderately severe plaque psoriasis and are clean, odourless and simple to apply.

Cautions

Use with caution in generalised pustular erythrodermic exfoliative psoriasis (BNF 2005).

Contraindications

Avoid in individuals with calcium metabolism disorders (BNF 2005).

Side effects

Local skin reactions, photosensitivity. Calcitriol is less irritant and can be used on the scalp and flexural areas. Rotational therapy (see below) is a useful strategy as tachyphylaxis can occur after a few weeks. This involves rotating vitamin D with other treatments every few weeks to ensure maximum benefit and efficacy.

Retinoids

Topical retinoids are useful in the management of mild to moderate plaque psoriasis although skin irritation is frequently reported. Care must be taken when applying onto specific psoriasis plaques in order to reduce the irritation of surrounding skin. Topical retinoids are not recommended for inflammatory psoriasis. Acitretin is a metabolite of Etretinate, a vitamin A derivative and is useful as a combination therapy with Ultraviolet Light (RUVA). This systemic retinoid is only available as a specialist treatment as careful monitoring is required (for a description of the mode of action, cautions, contraindication and side effects of retinoids see Chapter 4).

Topical corticosteroids

Anti-inflammatory agents are not generally suitable for the sole treatment of widespread chronic plaque psoriasis as tachyphylaxis (reduced efficacy of topical treatment with ongoing usage) and rebound is common. The use of topical corticosteroids can also cause psoriasis to become unstable, and precipitate generalised pustular psoriasis and erythodermic psoriasis. Topical corticosteroids treat inflammatory lesions by an immunological effect and vasoconstriction. Mild to moderately potent topical steroids can be useful for mild to moderate stable psoriasis if used in the short term. Mild topical steroids are also useful in treating specific sites such as the face and flexures. Potent steroids are specifically contraindicated in widespread plaque psoriasis although under specialist supervision can be used for specific sites such as palms of hands, soles of feet and scalp (BNF 2005).

Corticosteroid hormones are formed in the cortex of the adrenal glands. Corticosteroids have two effects: mineralocorticoid or glucocorticoid. Glucocorticoid effects include the maintenance of normal blood sugar levels and they assist the body to recover in times of injury or stress. Mineralocorticoid effects include controlling the balance between the water content and mineral salts in the body. Large amounts of corticosteroids in the body will suppress the activity of the immune system and produce an anti-inflammatory effect. This is the main reason for their therapeutic use.

Mode of action

Corticosteroids act by enzyme inhibition, suppressing the formation of prostaglandin and leukotriene inflammatory mediators. They also decrease histamine release from basophils. Their effect is therefore to suppress the inflammation and allergic/immune responses (Hopkins 1999).

Side effects

Side effects occur most frequently if an individual is receiving a potent or high dose of corticosteroid therapy or, if treatment is long term and systemic. Side effects include:

- hyperglycaemia and diabetes;
- protein catabolism leading to a loss of bone mass, muscle atrophy and paper thin skin;

- lypolysis which can lead to an alteration of subcutaneous fat distribution resulting in a 'moon-face' and 'buffalo-hump';
- increased susceptibility to infection;
- poor wound healing;
- oedema;
- increased blood pressure;
- hypernatraemia;
- hypokalaemia;
- hirsutism;
- allergic reactions;
- increased gastric acidity leading to an exacerbation of peptic ulcers (Galbraith *et al.* 1999).

Topical corticosteroids vary with regard to their potency (Henry 2001). The following indicates preparation potency:

Mildly potent	Moderately potent	Potent	Very potent
Hydrocortisone	Alclometasone	Beclomethasone	Halcinonide
	Clobetasone	Betamethasone	Clobetasol
	Fluocinonide	Diflucortolone	
	Fluocortolone	Desoxymethasone	
	Flurandrenolone	Fluocinonide	
	Halcinonide	Fluticasone	
		Mometasone	
		Triamcinolone	

Source: Henry (2001).

Mild and moderately potent topical corticosteroids are rarely associated with side effects. However, care must be taken if products are applied over a large surface, if an occlusive dressing is applied to the area, or, if the skin is damaged, as systemic absorption will be increased. Permanent changes to the skin will occur if potent corticosteroids are used in high concentrations over a prolonged period of time. Thinning of the skin and prominent blood vessels are the most common side effects. Therefore, if they are to be applied to the skin on the face, mild corticosteroids should only be prescribed. Rebound erythroderma (reddening of the skin) can occur if a treatment is stopped abruptly (Henry 2001).

Systemic immunomodulators

Systemic drugs which act on the immune system (i.e. ciclosporin, hydrox-yurea and methotrexate) are used to manage and control severe complicated psoriasis which has failed to respond to topical therapies. Blood dyscrasias, hepatic and renal toxicity are known side effects and therefore careful coun-selling and monitoring are required.

Rotational topical therapy

Sequential use (rotational use) of topical therapies is an important consideration when reducing the risk of tachyphylaxis (Callen *et al.* (2003)). Similar drug groups and different drug groups have been used in rotational therapy with good effect.

New biologics

New biological agents have recently been licensed for psoriasis, e.g. etanercept and efalizumab currently licensed in UK. These agents require subcutaneous or intravenous injection and are useful in the management of severe, recalci-trant psoriasis.

Specialist referral

The majority of patients managed within the community setting with mild to moderate psoriasis cope well. Home management is always the main aim for patients with support and encouragement from health professionals to main-tain and control the stability of the disease. Some patients will require spe-cialist referral. These include:

a. Patients whose psoriasis suddenly relapses and becomes unstable.
b. Patients who develop generalised pustular psoriasis.
c. Patients who develop erythodermic psoriasis.
d. Patients who have failed to respond to conventional therapy.
e. Patients who require medications prescribed by consultant dermatolo-gists, e.g. methotrexate, cyclosporin, retinoids and ultra violet A (UVA).
f. Patients who have delayed in seeking medical help early in the disease course.

g. Patients who have been referred too late by the general practitioner (GP). Patients referred within three years of disease onset fair better, both clinically and psychologically.

REFERENCES

BNF 46 (2005) London: British Medical Association and the Royal Pharmaceutical Society of Great Britain.

Callen JP, Krueger GG, Lebwohl M *et al.* (2003) AAD consensus statement on psoriasis therapies. *J Am Acad Dermatol* 49: 897–9.

Elder JT, Nair RP, Henseler T *et al.* (2001) The genetics of psoriasis 2001: the odyssey continues. *Arch Dermatol* 137: 1447–54.

Galbraith A, Bullock S, Manias E, Hunt B & Richards A (1999). *Fundamentals of Pharmacology.* London: Addison Wesley Longman Ltd.

Henry JA (2001) *The British Medical Association Concise Guide to Medicines and Drugs.* London: Dorling Kindersley.

Higgins E (2000) Alcohol, smoking and psoriasis. *Clin Exp Dermatol* 25: 107–10.

Hopkins SJ (1999) *Drugs and Pharmacology for Nurses.* Edinburgh: Churchill Livingstone.

Ingram JT (1953) The approach to psoriasis. *BMJ* ii: 591–4.

Koo J (1996) Population based epidermologic study of psoriasis with emphasis on quality of life assessment. *Dermatol Clin* 14: 485–96.

Leder RO, Mansbridge JN, Hallmayer J & Hodge SE (1998) Familial psoriasis and HLA–B: unambiguous support for linkage in 97 published families. *Hum Hered* 48: 198–211.

Mason AR, Cork MJ, Dooley G, Edwards G & Mason JM (2004) Topical Treatment for chronic plaque psoriasis (protocol). *The Cochrane Database of Systemic Reviews* Issue/Art.No:CD005028 D01: 10.1002/14651858.CD005028.

Nathan A (1997) Products for skin problems. *Pharmaceut J* 259 (6964): 606–10.

Rasmussen JE (2000) The relationship between infection with group A beta haemolytic streptococci and the development of psoriasis. *Pediatr Infect Dis* 19: 151–4.

Storbeck K, Holzle E, Schurer N *et al.* (1993) Narrow band UVB (311 nm) versus conventional broadband UVB with and without dithranol in phototherapy for psoriasis. *J Am Acad Dermatol* 28 (2): 227–31.

6

Eczema

Eczema or dermatitis is the most common inflammatory skin condition seen in primary care and accounts for approximately 30–40% of dermatology consultations (Williams 1997; Horn 1986; Steele 1984). Eczema affects both the dermis and the epidermis of the skin with numerous clinical presentations (see Tables 6.1 and 6.2). The commonest forms of eczema managed by primary care nurses are atopic eczema, hand eczema, contact dermatitis, asteototic eczema and gravitational eczema. The principles of treating all eczematous conditions are identical and will be discussed in this chapter.

Histopathology of eczema

The histology of eczematous skin shows spongiosis (intercellular epidermal oedema), vesicle formation (fluid accumulation), lymphocyte infiltration, acanthuses (thickening), parakeratosis (presence of superficial nucleated keratinocytes) and hyperkeratosis (thickening of the horny layer). Dermal changes include vasodilatation and leakage of blood cells (extravasation) into the surrounding tissues. This represents the inflammatory process of eczema (Bridgett *et al.* 1996) (see Figures 6.1–6.3).

These histological changes in the skin differ with the varying stages of the disease:

1. *Acute stage*: The changes in this stage include vasodilatation, extravasation (leaking blood cells into surrounding tissues) spongiosis, lymphocytic infiltration and vesicle formation over a period of hours and days.

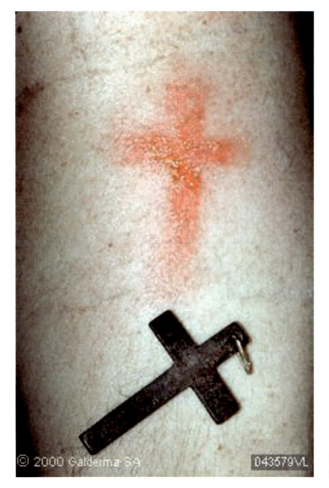

Fig. 6.1 Eczema contact.

2. *Subacute stage*: The changes in this stage include diminished vasodilatation, extravasation, lymphocytic infiltration, spongiosis, vesicle formation and increasing acanthosis and parakeratosis (over a period of days and weeks).

3. *Chronic stage*: Changes during this stage include acanthosis, parakeratosis, hyperkeratosis, dermal vasodilatation and extravasation over a period of weeks and months.

4. *Recovery and remission*: During this stage the histological changes return to normal if there are no secondary complications such as infection or trauma. This stage occurs over a period of weeks and months.

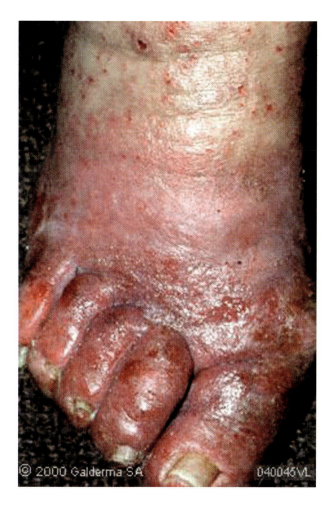

Fig. 6.2 Eczema infected.

5. *Relapse*: During relapse, acute episodes reoccur due to endogenous or exogenous triggers.

Clinical features

The clinical features of eczema relate specifically to the histological changes in the skin (Table 6.1).

Table 6.1 Histological changes and associated clinical features of eczema.

Stage	Histological changes	Clinical features
Acute (wet, weeping eczema)	Predominant epidermal spongiosis, vesicle formation, dermal vasodilatation, extravasation of blood cells, lymphocytic infiltration of epidermis	Red inflamed skin Superficial oedema Vesicle formation Vesicle rupture Exudate present Pruritus/pain Irritability/sleep loss Loss of function Loss of skin integrity
Subacute (wet/dry eczema)	Diminishing spongiosis, lymphocytic infiltration, vesicle formation, Increasing acanthosis, parakeratosis	Red/pink inflammation Vesicle/erosions Crusting drying exudate Scale formation Exfoliation Pruritus Irritability/sleep loss Loss of skin integrity
Chronic (Dry itchy eczema)	Predominant epidermal acanthosis, parakeratosis, hyperkeratosis, dermal vasodilatation and extravasation	Pink inflamed skin Dry, scaling skin hyperkeratosis Lichenification Pruritus

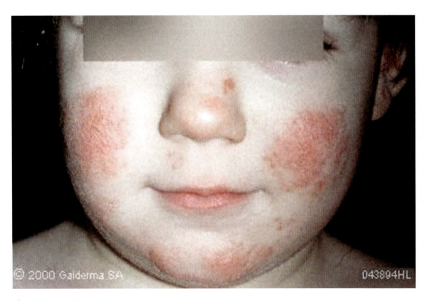

Fig. 6.3 Atopic eczema.

Table 6.2 Classification of eczema.	
Exogenous eczemas	Endogenous eczemas
• Contact eczema (allergic and photo-allergic)	• Atopic eczema
• Irritant eczema	• Seborrhoeic eczema
• PLE eczema	• Asteototic eczema
• Infective eczema	• Discoid eczema
	• Chronic scaly superficial dermatitis
	• Juvenile plantar dermatitis
	• Gravitational eczema (varicose)
	• Hand eczema
	• Drug eruptions
	• Pityriasis
	• Eczema associated systemic disease

Classification of eczema

Traditionally eczema is grouped into two categories: endogenous (from within) or exogenous (triggered by external factors) (Table 6.2).

Management principles

All the medical and nursing interventions for eczema are underpinned by the following principles:

- An understanding by patients and carers of the long-term relapsing nature of the disease, and the treatments available.
- The availability of psychosocial support from health professionals and patient support groups (e.g. National Eczema Society).
- A reduction in the exposure to 'trigger' factors (e.g. heat, humidity, foods, irritants such as water, soaps, detergents, wool, mineral oils, airborne allergens such as house dust mite, grasses and pollens, psychological factors such as stress).
- The application of emollients and anti-inflammatory agents.
- The treatment of complications (e.g. antibiotics for infections and anti-histamines or anti-pruritics for pruritus).

Assessment

Both eczema and psoriasis belong to the category of chronic inflammatory diseases which require ongoing physical and psychological assessment. Therefore, as psoriasis (see Chapter 5) a thorough and complete clinical assessment of the patient with eczema is required.

General history

- *Past medical history*: Age of patient. Age at onset of eczema. Past medical illnesses and operations, previous skin disease (especially in childhood or those triggered by infection), history of allergy or sensitivities, prescribed medications, over-the-counter medications, herbal remedies and vitamins. Child bearing potential, desire to impregnate, liver disease, hypertension, smoking and alcohol intake.
- *Family history*: Atopy eczema, psoriasis, autoimmune diseases, allergies, familial diseases.
- *Social history (essential in assessment of exogenous eczemas)*: Allergic contact eczemas, irritant eczema, polymorphic light eruption (PLE), photo- and phyto- (plant induced allergies) allergic eczemas.

  Occupation, leisure and sport interests, home situation, travel abroad, pets and animals. Potential trigger factors such as drugs, environment, stress, physical chemical or emotional trauma. Coincidental-related disease (e.g. HIV). The ability to access treatment (community-based and hospital-based services).

Physiological assessment

- *Clinical history of skin lesions and eczema development*:
  - Duration of eczema: How and when did eczematous lesions begin to appear?
  - How frequently has eczema appeared?
  - Presence and description of lesions.
  - What types of lesions are present? (Vesicles, exudates, scaling lesions, erythematous lesions, excoriations, crusting lesions, pustular lesions, lichenification, nodular lesions.)

- Site of eczematous lesions?
- Does anything make the eczema better or worse?
- Is the skin itchy or painful? (Evidence of excoriations, shiny fingernails from scratching and rubbing.)
- Localised or generalised lesions?
- *Distribution of lesions*:
  - Localised or generalised lesions?
  - Hand eczema, contact eczemas, gravitational eczema, asteototic eczema, juvenile plantar dermatoses, discoid eczema are all usually localised. Atopic eczema, drug eruptions and PLE can be generalised.
  - Hypo/hyper-pigmentation of skin or lesions (post-inflammatory residual hyper-pigmentation).
  - Presence of nail changes?

Psychological assessment

Quality of life considerations are important. These will include ability to perform activities of daily living, employability, interpersonal relationships. Psychological morbidity such as feelings of isolation, anxiety and depression is frequently reported in patients with severe eczema. Eczema sufferers can develop a low self esteem, which can impact on all aspects of the person's personal, social and working relationships.

- Psychological impact:
  Self concept (from the patient's perspective):
  - How does the skin appear to others?
  - How does the patient (and others) react to this?
  Self image:
  - How does the patient cope with the look of his/her skin?
  Concordance:
  - How has the patient coped with current/previous treatments?
  - What is the patient's understanding in relation to the disease, treatment and prognosis and are there any knowledge deficits? Patient's willingness in being involved in decisions about their skin treatments, previous satisfaction or dissatisfaction with treatments or progress.

If using a clinical and/or psychological assessment tool it is important to document serial measurements to assess progress and satisfaction. These tools can help reassure the patient that progress is being made, and also help reassure the health professional that referral to a specialist is appropriate.

It is important to include information from both the physiological and psychological assessments before categorising the severity of the eczema (i.e. mild, moderate or severe). 'Mild' localised eczema may still warrant secondary care referral if the patient's quality of life, activities and functioning has been affected. However, as a general rule of thumb, mild to moderate eczema is managed in primary care on a home management basis using topical therapies. Moderate to severe disease includes those patients with more than 5% body surface area (BSA) or those requiring more aggressive therapies such those who have lesions on the hands, soles, scalp and genitalia.

Preparation for treatment of eczema

The main groups of drugs used in the management of eczema are:

1. Emollients
2. Anti-inflammatory agents
3. Anti-infective agents.

Emollient therapies

Emollients represent the mainstay of treatment for eczema and can be prescribed as bath additives, soap substitutes and moisturises. All three formulations should be prescribed in any management plan and are used specifically to soothe, smooth and rehydrate the skin which enhances absorption of active treatments on the skin. Patient preference is far more important than professional choice when considering prescriptions for patients with eczema (Bridgett *et al.* 1996). Emollients also have a mild anti-inflammatory effect and if used appropriately can be steroid sparing (Holden *et al.* 2002). Numerous formulations are available ranging from aqueous based lotions and creams to greasier ointments and pastes. The vehicle is important to consider when using emollients for eczematous conditions. As rule of thumb 'the drier the skin the more greasy the emollient'. For example, chronic hyperkeratotic eczema will require an ointment for a greater therapeutic effect. Creams and water-based formulations are very short acting therefore requires frequent application to have the same therapeutic effect (see Chapter 5 'Psoriasis' for mode of action and contra-indications).

Anti-inflammatory agents for eczema

The main group of topical drugs prescribed for eczema (in primary care) for their anti-inflammatory action are the corticosteroids. These preparations are not curative and should be used intermittently. The newer immunosuppressive macrolides drugs (see Chapter 3) are regarded as second line treatment for atopic eczema and are usually prescribed initially by a dermatologist (National Prescribing Centre 2003).

Corticosteroids role in the management of eczema

Topical corticosteroids are available in varying potencies and are specifically indicated for use on the inflammatory component of eczema. Side effects, both local and systemic, are well documented and relate to topical use of moderately potent and potent steroids (BNF 2005). Therefore, it is important to titrate the dose and frequency of application of topical steroids to gain therapeutic effect and reduce the risk of side effects (see Chapter 5 for mode of action, contra-indications and side effects of topical corticosteroids).

Role of anti-infective agents in the management of eczema

Due to the nature of eczema secondary infection represents a clinical problem if not diagnosed and treated promptly. Widespread bacterial, fungal and viral infection can occur. The commonest causative organism is *Staphylococcus aureus*. Vaccinia and Herpes Simplex infection in eczema (eczema herpeticum) is regarded as a dermatological emergency and require urgent specialist referral. In primary care, prescribing anti-infective agents for bacterial infections is commonplace (see Chapter 3). There are concerns however, about the increasing evidence of anti-bacterial resistance in eczema which may be due to prescribing practices. Monk (2004) discusses the evidence and offers guidance on prescribing of anti-infective agents for eczema to reduce resistance. The Primary Care

Dermatology Society (2000) also has guidelines available for the management of atopic eczema. Key points include:

- Avoid long-term use of topical antibiotics (fusidic acid, mupirocin).
- Manage suspected localised infected eczema with other anti-infective agents (hydrogen peroxide cream, potassium permanganate, chlorhexidine creams, lotions and washes, aluminium acetate).
- Discontinue topical antibiotics if systemic antibiotics are prescribed (flucloxacillin, erythromycin).
- Ensure a minimum of 10–14-day course of systemic antibiotics for infected eczema (flucloxacillin, erythromycin).

Other treatments for eczema

Table 6.3 highlights other treatments that can be used in the treatment of eczema in conjunction with emollients, topical corticosteroids and anti-infective agents.

Specialist referral

The majority of patients managed within the community setting with mild to moderate eczema cope well. Home management is always the main aim for patients with support and encouragement from health professionals to maintain and control the stability of the disease. Some patients will require specialist referral. These include:

a. Patients whose eczema suddenly relapses and is unresponsive to topical treatment.
b. Patients who develop generalised secondary infection especially if herpes simplex is suspected (eczema herpeticum).
c. Patients who develop erythodermic exfoliative dermatitis.
d. Patients who have failed to respond to conventional therapy and would benefit cognitive behavioural management.
e. Patients who require medications prescribed by consultant dermatologists (e.g. immunomodulators, ultraviolet therapy).
f. Patients who have delayed in seeking medical help early in the disease course.
g. Patients who have been referred too late by the general practitioner. Patients with atopic eczema referred within 3 years of disease onset fair better, both clinically and psychologically.

Table 6.3 Treatments for eczema other than emollients and anti-inflammatory agents.

Treatment	Comments
Systemic anti-histamines (see Chapter 7)	May help reduce itch. Non-sedating products tried initially. Sedating anti-histamines nocté may aid sleep.
Gamma linoleic acid	Complementary remedy evening primrose oil taken as oral supplements inconclusive evidence on efficacy.
Occlusive paste bandages	Contain zinc oxide or ichthomol (fossilised fish tar). Applied for 3–7 days. Useful for limbs and lichenified areas of eczema. Anti-inflammatory, anti-pruritic and emollient effect.
Occlusive 'wetwrap' bandages Two layer tubular retention bandage (e.g. tubifast, comfifast, actifast). Warm wet bandage applied over emollients next to skin. Second dry layer of bandage applied over wet layer. Remains *in situ* for 12–24 h	Useful for acute inflammatory eczema. Applied for 12–24 h. Applied over emollients only to enhance moisturising effect. Not to be applied over topical corticosteroids unless under strict medical supervision. Anti-inflammatory, anti-pruritic and reduces trauma to skin from scratching.
Cognitive behavioural therapy	Useful technique for patients with atopic eczema. Helps break the scratch itch cycle through behaviour modification and habit reversal. Complements conventional therapies through a psychological behavioural approach (Bridgett *et al.* 1996).

REFERENCES

BNF 49 (2005) London: British Medical Association and Royal Pharmaceutical Society of Great Britain. *British National Formulary* 49 Chapter 13.4; pp. 561.

Bridgett C, Noren P & Staughton R (1996) *Atopic Skin Disease: A Manual for Practitioners.* Petersfield: Wrightson Biomedical Publishing Ltd. Chapter 1; pp. 9–10.

Holden C, English J, Hoare C, Jordan A, Kownacki S, Turnbull R & Staughton RCD (2002) Advised best treatment for the use of emollients in eczema and other dry skin conditions. *J Dermatol Treat* 13: 103–6.

Horn R (1986) The pattern of skin disease in general practice. *Dermatol Pract* Dec 14–19.

Monk B (2004) Avoiding antibiotic resistance in eczema. Practice Nurs 15(8): 384–7.

National Prescribing Centre (2003) Atopic eczema in primary care. *MeRec Bull* 14(1): 1–4.

Primary Care Dermatology Society (2000) Guidelines for the management of atopic eczema. Summary. www.pcds.org.uk/information%20Resource/Guide_ manatopic. asp (accessed 21 Dec 2004).

Steele K (1984) Primary dermatological care in general practice. *J Roy College Gen Pract* 34: 22–4.

Williams HC (1997) The epidemiologically based health need assessment reviews. In: Dermatology: Health Care Needs Assessment Second Series (Eds Stevens A & Raftery J Eds). Oxford: Oxford Radcliff Medical Press, pp. 26–7.

7

Urticaria and angio-oedema

Urticaria (also known as hives) is a common skin condition which affects the dermis. It manifests as macules (flat lesions) and weals (superficial oedema) on the skin which are frequently erythematous and itchy (Marks 1983) (see Figure 7.1). It is a transient condition, with lesions appearing and disappearing within a few hours (Schocket 1993). This reaction can occur on a daily basis and involve numerous lesions with flares lasting a few days to weeks. Chronic cases can last for months or years although approximately half of urticaria cases undergo spontaneous resolution within 6 months (Champion *et al.* 1969). The age of onset is variable and can first appear in both childhood and throughout adult life.

Angio-oedema can also be associated with urticaria and is recognised as a similar but deeper reaction, affecting the subcutaneous (SC) layer, deeper dermis and submucosal tissues (Grattan 2000) (see Figure 7.2). Urticaria and angio-oedema are classified according to the duration of the lesions and trigger factors (see Tables 7.1 and 7.2). Therefore careful history taking and clinical assessment are important.

Pathophysiology

The weal and flare reaction of urticaria is due to increased permeability of the skin capillaries and venules. A major mediator in the development of weals, flare (erythema) and itch is histamine which is released from skin mast cells. The histamine which is released targets the H_1 receptors in the skin to initiate such a response. Hence the role of antihistamines in the management of urticaria (BNF 2005). Other inflammatory cell mediators may also be involved which promote and sustain the weal and flare response (e.g. the release of cytokines from leukocytes).

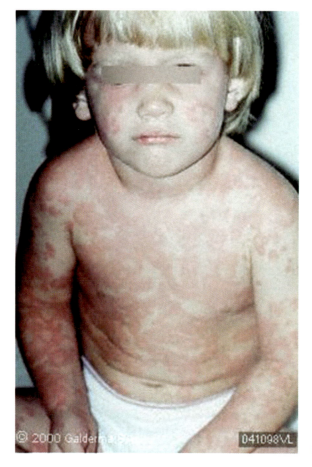

Fig. 7.1 Urticaria.

Non-allergic mast cell activation (and histamine release) can be triggered by neuropeptides (substance P), drugs (aspirin, morphine, codeine) and foods. Allergic mast cell activation initiates an immunological response involving IgE and release of histamine, and other mediators such as prostaglandins, leukotrienes, interleukins and cytokines (Black & Champion 1998).

Clinical presentation

During an acute onset, localised signs and symptoms include initial flat red lesions which progress to itchy raised weals anywhere on the skin including palms, soles of feet and scalp. These weals are characteristically surrounded by erythema (flare). Lesions vary in size shape and number and usually

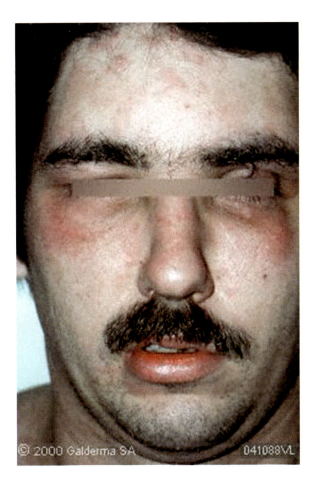

Fig. 7.2 Urticaria associated with angio-oedema.

resolve within 24 h leaving the skin with a normal appearance. Patients often do not realise the disappearance of individual lesions due to the vast numbers present. Frequently patients report urticaria as worse premenstrually and in the evening. Pruritus can be intense, leading to excoriations and bruising of the skin. Lesions in children can become purpuric. Angio-oedema is present in 50% of cases with clinical appearance of swollen lips, eyelids, oral cavity, tongue, larynx, pharynx, face in general, neck, arms, hands, feet and genitalia.

Systemic signs and symptoms

Urticaria and angio-oedema can be associated with general malaise, arthralgia, abdominal pain, gastrointestinal colic, dizziness, fainting, vomiting and

Table 7.1 Classification of urticaria and angio-oedema.

Classification	Comment
Ordinary urticaria (acute <6 weeks duration and chronic >6 weeks duration, episodic urticaria is intermittent acute activity)	(Clinical history excludes immune complex, physical and contact urticarias.) Chronic urticaria frequently termed idiopathic or autoimmune. Circulating auto-antibodies release histamine from mast cells. Triggers can be food additives (colourants), salicylates (aspirin), viral and bacterial infections and rarely inhalants (cigarette smoke, animal dander, pollens), menstrual cycle and pregnancy.
Physical and cholinergic urticarias	Triggers are physical: friction, stroking skin, pressure, cold contact, heat, aquagenic, exercise, sweating, sunlight.
Contact urticaria	Possible provocation by allergen and IgE mediated response.
Angio-oedema	Present without weals. Affects deeper tissues. May have hereditary C_1 esterase inhibitor deficiency. May be related to ACE inhibitors.
Immune complex urticaria	Serum sickness and urticarial vasculitis included in this group.
Other syndromes	Where urticaria is a component or condition and resembles angio-oedema and urticaria, for example, idiopathic oedema, systemic capillary leak syndrome, Schnitzler's syndrome, Muckle–Wells syndrome, Familial Mediterranean fever.

ACE: angiotensin-converting enzyme (*Source*: Black & Champion 1998).

diarrhoea. Analphylaxis with angio-oedema, hypotension and collapse has been reported as a severe systemic manifestation.

Psychological impact

Patients with urticaria, whether acute or chronic, frequently suffer sleep deprivation, fatigue and are highly embarrassed by the condition. Every aspect of their life may be adversely affected including working relationships, working

Table 7.2 Trigger substances.	
Acute allergic urticaria	Non-allergic urticaria
Bee and wasp stings	Drugs: penicillins, aspirin, NSAIDs
Drugs: penicillins, cephalosporins,	Plasma expanders
insulin, vaccines	Local anaesthetics
Blood products	General anaesthetics
Fish	
Shell fish (crab prawns, shrimp, lobster)	
Nuts	
Celery, beans potatoes, carrots, parsley	
Spices	
Fruits: bananas, apples oranges	
NSAIDS: non-steroidal anti-inflammatory drugs.	

abilities, personal relationships, self esteem, self-image resulting in psycho-logical morbidity (anxiety and depression) (Hashiro & Okumura 1990).

Assessment

General history

- Past medical history
  - Age of patient. Age at onset of urticaria. Past medical illnesses and operations, previous skin disease, especially in childhood or triggered by infection, diet, history of allergy or sensitivities, prescribed medications, over-the-counter medications, herbal remedies and vitamins. Child bearing potential, desire to impregnate, liver disease, hypertension, smoking and alcohol intake.
- Family history
  - Urticaria, angio-oedema, hereditary C_1 esterase inhibitor deficiency, urticarialvasculitis, atopy, eczema, autoimmune diseases, allergies, familial diseases.
- Social history
  - Occupation, leisure and sport interests, home situation, school situation, travel abroad, pets and animals. Sleep patterns. Potential trigger factors such as drugs, environment, stress, physical/chemical substance exposure.

Physiological assessment

- Clinical history of skin lesions
  Weal and flare development is important in order to confirm the diagnosis. Frequently, by the time the patient attends for consultations, there are no visible lesions on the skin, so it is important to ask about the following:
  - *Duration of urticaria episode*: How do they begin? How and when did weals/lesions begin to appear? How long do they last? Is there any redness associated with the weal? Do they disappear and reappear in a different place? How frequently do they appear? How long does it take for the entire rash to settle? Does the skin look normal after a flare up? Any associated facial swelling? Hands/feet swelling? Any associated breathing difficulties or wheezing? Any difficulties swallowing?
  - *Presence and description of lesions*: What types of lesions are present, that is, erythematous macules, papules, plaques annular lesions, serpintiginous lesions, linear lesions, excoriations, bruising, purpuric weals?
  - *The site of the eczematous lesions*: Body, face, scalp, groin?
  - Whether anything makes the urticaria better or worse?
  - Whether the lesions are itchy or painful?
  - Evidence of excoriations, shiny fingernails (from scratching and rubbing).
  - Hypo/hyper-pigmentation of skin or lesions (post-inflammatory residual hyper-pigmentation).
  - *Distribution of lesions*: localised or generalised lesions?
  - Transient lesions, that is, appearing, disappearing and reappearing at a different site.

Psychological assessment

Quality of life considerations are important. These will include ability to perform activities of daily living, employability, interpersonal relationships. Psychological morbidity such as feelings of isolation, anxiety and depression. Urticaria sufferers can develop a low self esteem, which can impact on all aspects of the person's personal, social and working relationships.

- Psychological impact
  - *Body image (from the patient's perspective)*: How does the skin appear to others? How does the patient (and others) react to this?
  - *Self esteem*: How does the patient cope with the look of his/her skin?
  - *Concordance*: How has the patient coped with current/previous treatments? What is the patient's understanding in relation to the disease,

treatment and prognosis and are there any knowledge deficits? Patient's willingness in being involved in decisions about their skin treatments. Previous satisfaction or dissatisfaction with treatments or progress.

Management of urticaria

Management is directed to control of symptoms rather than cure, and comprises general measures as well as medical intervention. Understanding the condition treatments and expected outcomes are essential for this group of patients. Therefore education, information, explanation and expectations help to reduce overall anxiety associated with the condition. It is important to inform the patient that the condition is not life threatening and will spontaneously resolve in about 50% of cases within 1 year (Lawlor 1998).

General measures

General measures involve *avoidance of identified triggers or reduced exposure to suspected trigger factors*:

- Avoid high risk over the counter analgesics and anti-inflammatory agents which contain aspirin, non-steroidal anti-inflammatory drugs (NSAIDs) or codeine. Substitute with paracetamol.
- Avoid prescription medicines known to aggravate urticaria, for example, angiotensin-converting enzyme (ACE) inhibitors.
- Minimise stress.
- Behaviour modification to avoid overheating and excessive exercise which induces sweating.
- Avoid foodstuffs which have a vasodilating effect, for example, alcohol, spices.
- Consider exclusion diet only if suspected triggers are in foods, for example, colourants, preservatives.

Emollient therapy

Application of emollients will help soothe the skin and is fundamental to dermatology management (see Chapter 5). Emollients with a soothing cooling antipruritic effect such as oily calamine lotion or cream, and aqueous cream with menthol 0.5–2%, are useful for itch. Emollient creams and lotions with antimicrobial action can promote healing of excoriated skin. Tepid baths and showers (low force) are advised.

Antihistamine therapy

First-line management for all patients with urticaria is systemic H_1 antihistamine therapy. The newer preparations, for example, acrivastine, cetirizine, loratdine, fexofenadine and terfenadine penetrate the blood–brain barrier to a lesser extent (causing less of a sedatory effect) are the drugs of choice.

Mode of action

Antihistamines compete with histamine (released from mast cells) and block its action at histamine receptor sites in the skin, blood vessels, nasal passages and airways.

Side effects

Drowsiness, headaches, dulling of mental alertness and antimuscarinic effects (e.g. dry mouth, blurred vision, urinary retention, gastrointestinal disturbances) are all greatly reduced with the newer antihistamines. Other side effects include palpitations and arrhythmias (this is especially associated with terfenadine).

Second-line long-term therapy using systemic steroids (see Chapter 5) is not recommended for urticaria. These preparations may be considered in specific cases where short-term therapy (3 days to 3 weeks) is required for vascular urticaria, or as a stat dose to reduce laryngeal oedema and prevent anaphylaxis. Topical steroids are ineffective for urticaria. Epinephrine (intramuscular (IM)/subcutaneous (SC) injection) is indicated as an emergency drug in the event of anaphylaxis and severe laryngeal/pharyngeal oedema.

When to refer for specialist opinion

Urticaria can be a difficult condition to control and referral to a dermatologist is advised when:

- Patients do not respond to first-line management and patient concordance is confirmed.
- Patients requires specific tests and investigation, for example, full blood count, physical challenge tests, exercise tests, cold challenge tests, skin biopsy.

- Patients are suspected of C_1 esterase inhibitor deficiency.
- Patients with suspected urticarial vasculitis require a skin biopsy.
- Further differential diagnosis is required, for example, Polymorphic Light Eruption (PLE), pemphigoid.
- Severe there is acute exacerbation with angio-oedema.
- The psychological impact of disease warrants specialist assessment and intervention.

REFERENCES

BNF 49 (2005) British Medical association and Royal Pharmaceutical Society of Great Britain. British National Formulary 49 Chapter 13.4.1; pp. 159–63.

Black AK & Champion RH (1998) Urticaria. In: *Textbook of Dermatology* (Eds Champion RH, Burton JL, Burns DA & Breathnach SM) 6th edn. Oxford: Blackwell Scientific. Vol 3, Chapter 47; pp. 2113–39.

Champion RH, Roberts SOB, Carpenter RG & Roger JH (1969) Urticaria and angio-oedema: a review of 554 cases. *Br J dermatol* 81: 558–97.

Grattan CEH & Francis DM. (2000) Autoimmune urticaria. In: *Advances in Dermatology* 15, St Louis Mosby Inc.

Hashiro M & Okumura M (1990) Anxiety, depression, psychomotor symptoms and autonomic nervous function in patients with chronic urticaria. *J Dermatol Science* 123: 129–35.

Lawlor F (1998) Diagnosing and treating common urticaria. *Dermatol Pract.* May/June: 18–20.

Marks R (1983) *Practical Problems in Dermatology London Martin Dunitz Ltd.* Chapter 32; pp. 205–10.

Schocket AL (Ed.) (1993) *Clinical Management of Urticaria and Anaphylaxis.* New York: Marcel Dekker.

8

Infections and infestations of the skin

Infections of the skin are frequently seen in primary care. The causative organisms are usually bacterial, viral or fungal.

Bacterial skin infections

The most common skin infection is usually caused by a pathogenic organism which has colonised the skin. *Staphylococcus* and streptococcus are the most commonly seen pathogens and are responsible for a variety of skin infections.

Impetigo

Impetigo is a highly infectious superficial skin infection, commonly seen in children, which can quickly spread to other members of the family or persons in close skin contact (see Figure 8.1). The causative organism is usually *Staphylococcus aureus* or a β-haemolytic streptococcus. Impetigo appears as localised lesions of inflamed patches which are covered in a yellow crust. Common sites are the face, limbs and hands. The blistering form of impetigo (bullous impetigo) appears as fluid filled lesions. These lesions quickly rupture to form erosions which then develop yellow crusting. Occasionally the bullous form can be severe with blood filled (haemorrhagic) lesions. Secondary bacterial infection of skin conditions such as infestations, eczema, cold sores (herpes simplex) can frequently become impetiginised (British Association of Dermatologists (BAD) 2005).

Assessment

Clinical assessment involves:

- Distribution and duration
- History of previous infections

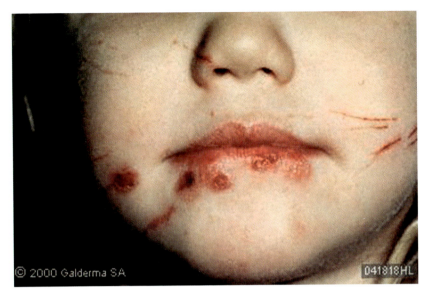

Fig. 8.1 Impetigo.

- History of diabetes mellitus
- $+/-$ general malaise upon onset
- Family history
- Type of lesion:
  - presence of yellow crusting
  - underlying erythema
  - bullous form: Fluid filled blisters (clear, yellow, haemorrhagic)
  - bullous form: Erosions with yellow crusting

Treatment

Treatment always includes:

- General skin care advice:
  - avoid sharing face cloths, sponges, towels, etc.
  - gentle washing and removal of crusts using mild antimicrobial emollients (Dermol range) (see Chapter 5) including a soap substitute or moisturiser and disposable wipes.
- Appropriate topical antibiotic therapy (localised infections)
  - Mupirocin
  - Fuscidic acid

- Systemic antibiotic therapy if severe or widespread
  - Flucloxacillin
  - Erythromycin
  - Benzyl penicillin (streptococcal infections)

(See Chapter 3 for antibacterial therapy)

Folliculitis

Folliculitis is an infection of the hair follicles usually caused by the staphylo-coccus bacterium. Folliculitis appears as multiple, superficial, erythematous lesions with a central pustule. Typical skin sites are the thighs, legs, buttocks and face. Discomfort can be experienced although more often, folliculitis is asymptomatic. Incorrect application of emollients (especially greasy prepar-ations) can precipitate folliculitis. To prevent this, emollients and moisturisers should not be rubbed into the skin. Application on the skin in the direction of the hair growth helps avoid plugging and clogging of the hair follicles which precipitates folliculitis.

Boils (furuncle and carbuncle)

A furuncle (boil) is a deeper acute folliculitis and can be extremely painful. Furuncles can appear as isolated or multiple lesions which can be localised or widespread. They appear on the skin as raised erythematous lesions which develop into pustule. These frequently ruptures and releases pus. Boils can spontaneously resolve. However, due to the pain and tenderness experienced, many people seek medical advice for surgical lancing and antibiotic therapy which hasten recovery. The term carbuncle is used when numerous furuncles coalesce resulting in a large painful erythematous nodular lesion with mul-tiple pustules on the skin surface. The causative organism is *S. aureus* which thrives in areas of the skin which are moist such as the axilla, groin and scalp. These harbour sites are frequent sites for boils, although, they can occur anywhere on the skin (BAD 2005).

Treatment
Treatment always includes:

- General skin care advice:
  - avoid sharing face cloths, sponges, towels, etc.
  - gentle washing

- clean hands and short nails
- avoid touching and squeezing lesions (unless under medical supervision for lancing)
- use mild antimicrobial emollients as cleansers/moisturisers and disposable wipes
- frequent washing of clothing at recommended temperature
- avoid obesity (germ harbours in folds of skin)
- Topical antibiotic or antiseptics
  - Clorhexidene washes to skin
  - Iodine washes to skin
  - Antiseptic bath additives containing triclosan
  - Antibiotic ointment in nostrils (3 times daily for 10 days)
  - Consider treating other nasal carriers within family
- Systemic antibiotic therapy if severe, widespread or recurrent (minimum 10-day course) (see Chapter 3)
  - Flucloxacillin
  - Erythromycin

Chronic paronychia

Paronychia is a localised bacterial infection of the nail fold or cuticle The causative organism is usually *S. aureas*. The fungal yeast candida albicans can also be involved (see Figure 8.2). The lesion appears as a painful red shiny swelling in or around the skin of the nail fold (Gillespie & Bamford 2000). The inflammation spreads around the cuticle and separates the skin away from the nail plate. Localised oedema is apparent with exudates of pus on palpation. Chronic paronychia is the term used when the infection continues for more than 6 weeks. A brownish black or green discolouration and ridges may be seen in the nail. Those most at risk of developing chronic paronychia are (BAD 2005):

- Females, especially those who have frequent cuticle manicures (skin integrity becomes broken).
- Workers involved in wet hand work with detergents (e.g. bakers kitchen aids, bar attendants, housewives).
- Individuals with a history of diabetes mellitus.
- Individuals with a history of recurrent thrush infection.
- Persons with poor peripheral circulation to hands and feet.

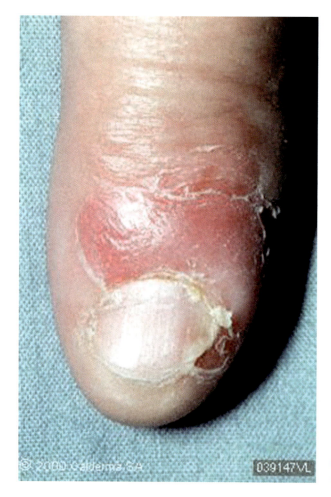

Fig. 8.2 Nail candidiasis.

Assessment

Clinical assessment involves:

- Duration and distribution of lesion or infection
- Onset of this infection
- History of previous infections (fungal as well as bacterial)
- History of diabetes mellitus
- +/− general malaise upon onset
- Family history
- Occupational/social history
- Skin swab for microbiology and mycology

General advice
- Reduce or avoid wet work with detergents
- Wear cotton lined protective gloves
- Keep hands warm and dry
- Gentle washing/cleansing using antimicrobial emollients
- Avoid biting nails
- Avoid aggressive manicures to cuticle

Treatment
- Topical antibiotics (see Chapter 3)
  - mupirocin
  - fusidic acid
- Systemic antibiotics (see Chapter 3)
  - flucloxicillin
  - erythromycin

Infected eczema

Infected eczema is usually due to a secondary *S. aureus* infection (see Chapter 6 for a comprehensive review of infected eczema).
- Topical antifungals
  - amorolfine cream
  - clotrimazole cream
  - fluconazole
- Systemic antifungals
  - fluconazole

Antifungal preparations

Mode of action
Antifungal agents interfere with fungal cell permeability, leading to prevention of cell replication and cell death.

Contraindications
The contraindications for fluconazole, miconazle are hepatic impairment and previous hypersensitivity to the drug. These preparations should be used with caution in pregnancy. It increases the activity of some other drugs when taken at the same time. These include anticoagulants (warfarin), antidiabetics (sulphonylureas) and antiepileptics (phenytoin). Miconazole

antagonises the effects of amphotericin. The only contraindication for the use of nystatin is a previous history of allergic reaction on exposure to the drug.

Caution – Terbinafine cream (Lamisil) – contact with eyes should be avoided. Caution should be taken if pregnant or breastfeeding.

Side-effects

Fluconazole may cause nausea, abdominal discomfort, flatulence, diarrhoea, liver function abnormalities, angioedema and anaphylaxis. Amorolfine and clotrimazole can cause occasional local irritation and hypersensitivity reactions. These include mild burning sensations, erythema and itching. Discontinuation of treatment is recommended (British National Formulary (BNF) 2005) if these occur.

Systemic adverse effects of topical preparations are rare as drug absorption is only slight. However, they can include a diuretic effect, abdominal cramping and local irritation. Lamisil may cause skin to become red and itchy.

Erysipelas and cellulitis

Erysipelas and cellulitis are deeper infections of the skin usually caused by streptococcus pyogenes infection (Gillespie & Bamford 2000). Generalised fever and malaise always precede the development of skin lesions. Erythematous, painful, oedematous patches appear on the skin. The affected skin is hot to touch, shiny in appearance and frequently has a 'stepped' edge or border. Erysipelas is a severe acute infection which commonly affects the face and can be accompanied by marked oedema of the peri-orbital region.

Cellulitis (see Figure 8.3) can occur anywhere in the deeper layers of the skin. Common sites include lower limb and face. The portal of entry for the streptococcus is usually due to a breakdown in skin integrity. A superficial cut, insect bite or athletes foot can be an entry site for the organism (BAD 2005). Recurrent cellulitis is a combination of a low-grade chronic condition with acute exacerbations. This is due to the organism lying dormant within the lymphatic system. Therefore it is important that appropriate antibiotic therapy is initiated and completed.

Assessment
- Details of onset, duration and distribution
- History/evidence of fever and malaise

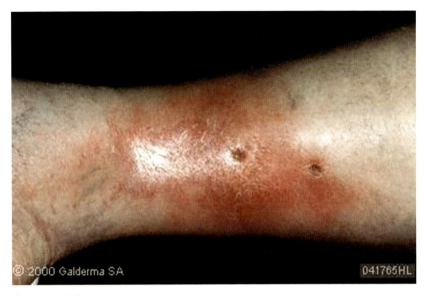

Fig. 8.3 Cellulitis.

- History of diabetes mellitus
- History of recurrent cellulitis
- Evidence of breakdown in skin integrity for example, insect bite, athletes foot, cut or abrasion
- Evidence of erythema, heat and oedema
- Skin shiny and hot to touch
- Skin swab obtained for microbiology

Treatment

Erysipelas and cellulitis are always treated with systemic antibiotic therapy (see Chapter 3). Cellulitis requires long-term systemic antibiotic therapy (minimum duration 1 month). The antibiotic of choice is benzyl penicillin (see Chapter 3).

General skin care advice

- avoid sharing face cloths, sponges, towels, etc.
- gentle washing using mild antimicrobial emollients including a soap substitute or moisturiser
- treat and heal any breakdown in skin integrity (e.g. athletes foot between toes webs)

When to refer a patient with suspected bacterial skin infections

Urgent referral for specialist opinion is required if there is:

- Widespread and severe skin infection
- Localised skin infections associated with hyperpyrexia and malaise
- Localised skin infections that has failed to respond to conventional treatment
- Sudden deterioration in skin integrity, development of bullae, haemorrhagic lesions
- Suspected superimposed viral infection

Viral skin infections

Benign warts

Warts and verrucae (plantar warts) (see Figure 8.4) are the most commonly seen viral infections on the skin. Human papilloma virus is the causative organism of which there are many types. Warts infect the cornified stratified squamous epithelium or the uncornified mucous membranes. They are contagious and can occur anywhere on the skin. Common sites include hands, fingers, soles of feet, knees and face. Clinical types include common warts, plane warts, plantar warts, mosaic warts, ano-genital warts, myrmecia (burrowing warts), intermediate warts and oral warts (Sterling *et al.* 2001).

Warts appear as flesh coloured or greyish coloured lesions. They are usually hyperkeratotic, raised nodules on the skin. Plane warts appear as raise smooth papules, usually seen on the face and hands. They can occur in isolation or in groups. Verrucae tend to be flat lesions which can develop areas of callous on weight bearing regions of the foot.

General skin care advice

- Avoid sharing of wash cloths, towels, etc.
- Daily paring down lesions with pumice stone or emeryboard following bath/shower
- Wash hands after touching warts or verrucae
- Wear protective swim socks if evidence of verrucae on feet
- Daily change of socks
- Daily rotation of shoes if possible

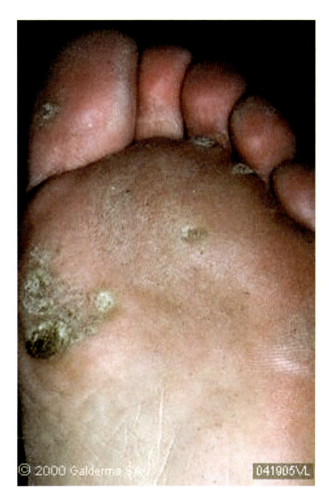

Fig. 8.4 Mosaic plantar warts.

Assessment

– Not all warts need treatment
– Indicators for treatment include pain, loss of function, embarrassment risk of malignancy
– Success rate of treatments: 60–70% clearance in 3 months
– Best success if treatment initiated sooner rather than later
– An immune response needs to be initiated before clearance occurs
– Immuno-compromised patients are at risk of multiple recalcitrant warts
– Persons with diabetes mellius are more at risk of developing viral warts and verrucae

– Warts are usually self limiting with spontaneous resolution occurring within 2–3 years
– Verrucae are more deeply embedded in the skin and can be persistent

Treatments
– Topical paints and lacquers offer limited results and have to be applied daily for minimum of 3 months
– Salicylic acid (a keratolytic) containing products (see Chapter 4)
– Topical retinoids (0.05% tretinoin cream) (see Chapter 4)

• Paring down of lesions following bathing and before treatment aids absorption of topical paints and lacquers
• Liquid Nitrogen (cryotherapy) can be performed at 3–4 weekly intervals for four to six sessions as per local protocol. Lesions should be pared down prior to freezing. Cryotherapy is a painful procedure and can result in scaring if performed aggressively.
• Other treatments
    – Photodynamic therapy (see Chapter 9)
    – Bleomycin
    – Formaldehyde
    – Thermocautery
    – Chemical cautery
    – Laser therapy
    – Topical desensitisation
    – Oral Cimetidine therapy salicylic acid (Sterling *et al.* 2001)

Molluscum contagiosum

Molluscum contagiosum are small round pearly papular lesions with evidence of a central crater or punctum. These benign lesions are caused by the pox virus and a commonly seen in children. Molluscum are self-limiting with spontaneous resolution within 6–18 months. They are, however, contagious and can quickly spread to siblings within the same family. Mollusucum can appear as single or multiple lesions anywhere on the skin and can be associated with an eczematous reaction in the surrounding skin. Common sites are the face, axilla, ano-genital area and trunk. Children with atopic eczema appear to be more prone to molluscum and it is linked with regular topical corticosteroid use. Molluscum can become impetiginised due to concurrent eczema, scratching and subsequent infection (BAD 2005).

General skin care advice

- Avoid sharing face cloths, sponges and towels
- Avoid bathing affected children together in the same bath
- Gentle bathing and cleansing using antimicrobial emollients
- Avoid scratching lesions as this will encourage spread to other sites
- Encourage hand hygiene following toilet
- Avoid contact sports and swimming
- Children can attend school

Treatment

- No specific treatment is required for molluscum contagiosum
- Topical antibiotic cream ($+/-$ steroid) can be applied to inflamed or infected lesions (see Chapter 3)
- Trauma to the lesions (picking, scratching, squeezing) will destroy the virus but can be painful for young children. Further spread may be encouraged if lesions are picked and scratched
- Wart paints can be applied to lesions (excluding those near the eyes)
- Topical immunomodulator cream can be applied (not in pregnancy)
- Liquid nitrogen (cryotherapy) can be used to treat individual or larger lesions but this is painful and distressing to most young children. A local anaesthetic cream can be applied prior to cryotherapy as a method of pain relief
- Curettage can be performed to larger lesions. However, this is painful and requires topical anaesthetic cream prior to the procedure.

When to refer

Generally warts and verrucae can be managed at home or within primary care services. Patients may require referral if:

- There is evidence of widespread, severe or disabling warts/verrucae unresponsive to long-term topical therapies and cryotherapy
- Immuno-compromised patients with widespread, severe or disabling warts, verrucae or molluscum
- Lesions present around the eye should be referred to an eye specialist

Herpes simplex virus and herpes zoster (shingles)

There are more than 80 herpes viruses of which eight affect humans. The most common of these are herpes simplex (HSV-I; HVS-II), varicella zoster virus (VZV),

Cytomegalvirus (CMV) and Epstien–Barr virus (EBV) (Clarke 2004). The most commonly seen viral infections in the community are herpes simplex (cold sore) and VZV (shingles).

The cold sore virus (HSV Type I, see Figure 8.5) usually occurs as a secondary recurrent infection on the skin. The virus can lie dormant in the sensory nerve ganglion of the spinal cord. When reactivated the virus then transfers along the nerve to the skin to produce the characteristic lesions. It can appear anywhere on the skin with common sites being the face, lips and mucous membranes (e.g. nostrils, vulva). The virus is transferred by touch (skin, mouth and sexual contact) and can be precipitated by ultraviolet radiation

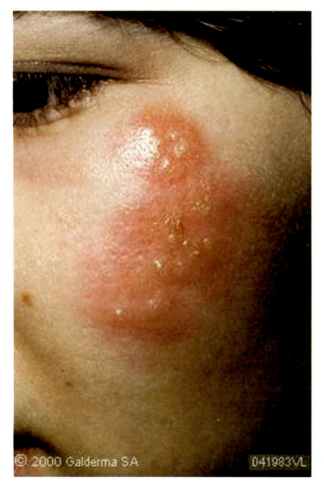

Fig. 8.5 Herpes simplex.

(sunshine), hormonal changes (premenstrual) and fever, infection or general malaise (stress). HSV infection is always associated with a preceding tingling, burning painful sensation on the skin site. This occurs prior to the eruption of fluid filled vesicles. Erythema and pain are always present during the first 48 hours of HSV infection. The vesicles eventually rupture with presence of exudate which dries and crusts. The healing process usually occurs within 7 days with no scaring. (BAD 2005).

HSV Type II is responsible for genital herpes, a painful and distressing condition during acute episodes. Type II herpes infection does not usually occur on other skin sites.

Anyone with active herpes infection should take care to reduce or avoid contact with at risk persons such as pregnant women, nursing mothers and children/babies with atopic eczema.

Herpes zoster (shingles – see Figure 8.6) is an acute infection caused by the VZV (chickenpox). Following a chicken pox infection the virus can lie dormant within the sensory nerve ganglion and be re-activated in later life. The reactivated viral infection appears on the skin as shingles (herpes zoster infection). As with HSV, onset is sudden with preceding pain or tingling of the affected skin. Zoster is always unilateral and blistering lesions follow dermatomes of the skin (e.g. the trigeminal nerve). Neuralgia is common following herpes

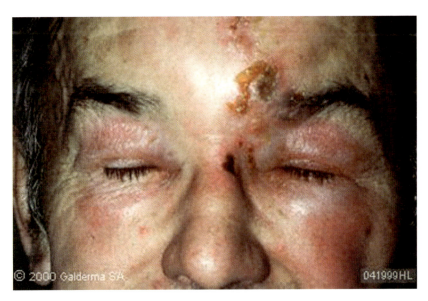

Fig. 8.6 Herpes zoster.

zoster infection and can be reduced if treatment is initiated early (i.e. prior to eruption of vesicles (BAD 2005)).

Assessment

Suspected HSV or HZV infection requires the following assessment:

- Onset and distribution of lesions
- History of tingling, pain over affected site
- History of fever or malaise
- History of diabetes mellitus
- History of previous HSV infection, Chicken Pox infection or shingles infection/post herpetic neuralgia
- Evidence of vesicles, erosions and crusting
- Family history/partner history
- Occupation
- Pregnancy

General advice

- Gentle cleansing of the area and bathing using antimicrobial emollients
- Cool compress and application of petroleum jelly to lesion site
- Avoid direct skin contact with others when lesions present
- Initiate treatment during early stages of development (before development of vesicles)
- Avoid direct contact with pregnant women, nursing mothers and babies
- Avoid direct contact with all persons, especially children, with atopic eczema
- Avoid direct skin contact with the elderly and the infirm
- Avoid direct skin contact with immuno-compromised people
- Avoid triggers which reactivate virus (e.g. sunburn, stress, becoming rundown)
- keep healthy and ensure adequate sleep

Treatment

- Antiviral drugs are always indicated for HSV and HZV infections
    - Aciclovir
    - Famciclovir
    - Valaciclovir
- Localised mild infections may be treated with topical application
    - Aciclovir
    - Famciclovir

- Moderate/severe/widespread or recurrent infections require systemic anti-viral treatment
  - Aciclovir
  - Famciclovir
  - Valaciclovir
- Analgesia
  - during an active infection
  - post herpetic neuralgia may require ongoing analgesia
- Antibiotics (see Chapter 3)
  - if secondary bacterial infection suspected (Impetiginised)
- Rest
  - reduces stress, hastens recovery

Antiviral treatment

Mode of action
Aciclovir, famciclovir and valaciclovir are antiviral preparations. These substances work by inhibiting viral DNA replication. They compete with viral substrates to form ineffective DNA chains. Although the virus is not eradicated and can reoccur, its multiplication is prevented. Spread of the virus to uninfected cells is stopped and symptoms improve (Galbraith *et al.* 1999).

Caution
Renal impairment, pregnancy and breastfeeding.

Side effects
Nausea, vomiting, abdominal pain, headache, fatigue, rash, photosensitivity.

When to refer

Urgent referral to hospital is required if:

- Widespread severe herpes infection (unresponsive to treatment)
- Evidence of infection in or near eye(s) requires referral to an eye specialist
- Suspected herpes infection in atopic eczema (Eczema Herpeticum)
- Development of fever, malaise, severe pain
- Evidence of secondary bacterial infection (impetiginised)
- Active severe herpes infection during pregnancy (first and last trimester most at risk)

Fungal infections

Fungal infections can be caused by yeast, moulds and dermatophytes.

Dermatophyte infections (*Tinea* or ringworm)

There are three genera of dermatophytes: Trichophyton, Microsporum and Epidermophytum. Skin and nail (onychomychosis – see Figure 8.7) infections involving dermatophytes are frequently referred to as *Tinea* infections or ringworm (Volk 1982).

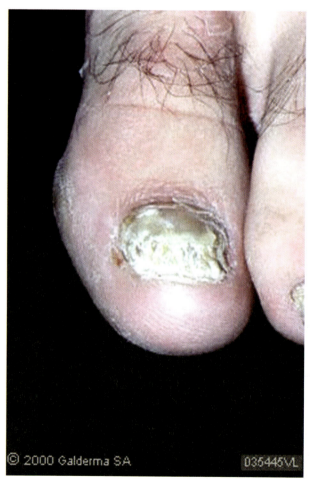

© 2000 Galderma SA   035445VL

Fig. 8.7
Onychomycosis.

- *Tinea pedis*   Ringworm of foot
- *Tinea coroporis* Ringworm of body
- *Tinea capitis*   Ringworm of scalp
- *Tinea cruris*   Ringworm of groin
- *Tinea unguium*   Ringworm of the nails
- *Tinea manuum*   Ringworm of the palms
- *Tinea barbae*   Ringworm of the beard area

Tinea pedis (athletes foot) is a commonly seen dermatophyte infection, usually present in the toe webs. *Tinea unguium* (Onychomychosis) affects the nail and can co-exist with *Tinea pedis* in toe webs and candida infection or *Tinea manuum* of the fingers and hands. *Tinea corporis* can occur anywhere on the skin and is usually seen on the limbs and trunk. *Tinea manuum* affects the palms of the hands and fingers. *Tinea capitis* is scalp ringworm manifesting as red scaly patches with hair loss. It is predominantly seen in children (particularly the Afro-Caribbean population) and can be widespread in urban areas. *Tinea capitis* can present as a persistent scaly scalp in young children. Skin scrapings and hair samples should be obtained for mycology to exclude the possibility of fungal infection (Higgins *et al.* 2000). *Tinea capitis* can develop into kerion, a chronic severe pustular condition if untreated.

All Ringworm infections can be acquired from contact with other humans, animals or from objects and soil.

Assessment

Fungal infections can become widespread and severe if left untreated or treated inappropriately. Therefore assessment should include skin scrapings and/or nail clippings for mycological examination if in any doubt as to the diagnosis.

Misdiagnosis can lead to inappropriate treatment as is seen in the condition *Tinea* incognita which occurs due to application of topical corticosteroids to ringworm infection. The application of the steroid masks the clinical appearance of ringworm by reducing erythema and scaling. The fungal growth itself is unaffected by steroids and the infection persists and spreads.

Assessment also includes:

- Sites, onset, duration and distribution of lesions
- Signs and symptoms associated with infection
- Current treatment

- Previous treatments
- History or previous infections
- History of diabetes mellitus
- Past medical history (immuno-compromised)
- Family history of infection
- Social interests and occupation
- Skin scrapings/nail clippings/hair samples for mycology depending on site of infection

Candidiasis

Yeasts are responsible for candidal infections seen on the skin, especially around nail folds, mucous membranes, perineal and interiginous regions and areola.

Classical oral candidisis (thrush) can spread via the alimentary canal to the ano-genital area especially in babies. Oral thrush appears a white creamy substance overlying erythematous lesions on the tongue and mucous membranes.

Angular chelitis may also be aggravated by a candidal infection. This appears as persistent erythematous lesions or fissures at the corners of the mouth and lips. This is frequently an ongoing problem in the elderly, who, on further examination have dentures and are harbouring an oral thrush infection.

Simple intertrigo is an eczematous skin reaction of the flexures, where two skin surfaces touch (Marks 1983). These areas can become infected with candida. Common sites are the axillae, under breasts, folds of abdominal skin, inner thighs, between buttocks and groin area. The infection appears as large patches of erythema, frequently with a shiny surface. There may be the presence of white scaling at the outer edge or border of the lesion(s).

Candidiasis of the groin area may include the mucous membranes of the vulva and vagina with skin involvement extending over the labia, mons pubis, inner thigh and perineum. Satellite lesions of erythematous papules or pustules are commonly seen surrounding the larger patches. A similar distribution and presentation is seen in infants throughout the nappy area.

Candidal infections can also occur in the male genitals affecting predominantly the glans and the neck of the penis and extend over the scrotal skin to the inner thigh and perineal skin.

Intertrigo and groin/genital candidal infections can be intensely itchy and painful.

Assessment

Assessment will include clinical examination of all skin harbour sites including oral cavity, axillae, intertriginous areas, groin and nail beds/cuticles.

- Site, onset, duration and distribution of rash
- Types of lesions
- Symptoms
- Previous history of fungal infections
- History of diabetes mellitus
- Previous treatments (unjudicial use of topical steroids)
- Contacts and partners
- Skin swab taken for mycology

Treatment of fungal infections

Fungal infections are always treated with:

- Antifungal/anti-yeast agents for skin infection (topical)
  - amorolfine cream
  - terbinafine cream
  - clotrimazole cream
  - miconazole nitrate cream
  - ketoconazole cream
  - econazole nitrate cream
  - fluconazole cream
  - nystatin cream
  - benzoyl peroxide cream
  - benzoic acid ointment
  - sulconazole nitrate cream
  - undecenoates paint, cream, powder, sprays
- Antifungal/anti-yeast agents for nail infection (topical)
  - Amorolfine nail lacquer
  - Tioconazole nail solution
  - Salicylic acid paint
- Combination antifungal/antibacterial agents (topical)
  - miconazole nitrate/hydrocortisone cream/ointment
- Systemic antifungals if widespread and or internal
  - terbinafine
  - itraconazole
  - nystatin
  - griseofulvin (licensed for use in children)

(see chronic paronychia for the mode of action, contraindications, adverse effects for antifungal agents)

Topical corticosteroids are not indicated as a monotherapy

General skin care advice

- Gentle cleansing and bathing using antimicrobial emollients
- Avoid sharing wash cloths, towels, nail clippers, etc.
- Gentle drying of moist skin areas especially between toes
- Avoid over-heating and sweating
- Avoid use of talcum powder to intertriginous areas
- Cool cotton clothing worn between skin surfaces
- Avoid obesity
- Persons with diabetes mellitus are at risk of secondary super infections

Nail care

- Regular foot and nail care, including cleansing, drying and clipping (use 2nd pair of clippers for infected toe nails)
- Use an antifungal cream for toe webs and surrounding skin, as well as a nail preparation for onychomycosis
- Do not delay treatment. Commence topical treatments when infection first noticed
- Regular change of socks and footwear
- Wear 'breathable' footwear whenever possible
- Wear protective socks, flip-flops, sandals in communal swimming pools, locker rooms and shower rooms

When to refer

- Widespread severe infection unresponsive to topical therapies
- Severe infection with secondary infection
- Severe or troublesome infection in at risk patients (e.g. immuno-compromised patients, elderly and infirm, infants and babies).

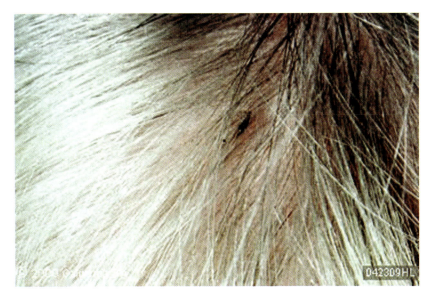

Fig. 8.8 Head lice.

Infestations of the hair and skin

Lice

Parasitic lice commonly infest human skin and hair. They are transferred by direct contact and can live happily on all types of skin and hair. The stigma attached to lice relates to a lack of cleanliness as body lice were mainly seen on vagrants, the homeless and soldiers at war. Body lice can live on clothing, particularly the seams, and thus were common in persons who did not have the opportunity to wash and change clothes frequently. Pubic lice (crabs) are transferred by sexual contact and is common in young adults. Scalp Lice (see Figure 8.8) are also associated with a lack of cleanliness but experience has shown that head lice can, and do, infest clean heads. Much of the education and management of lice deals with reducing the stigma surrounding lice to effect adequate management. Lice are live, six legged parasites which lay eggs (nits) on the shaft of hairs. An infestation of lice can cause intense itching and scratching due the skin's reaction to lice bites, saliva and excrement. Scratching can lead to excoriation which in turn can become secondarily infected (impetiginised) (Lachapelle *et al.* 1994).

Pediculosis capitis (head lice) is the commonest form of infestation seen in the UK. It can affect anyone but, particularly children aged between 4–11. The lice are transferred by head-to-head contact or occasionally by sharing of combs, hats and pillows. (BAD 2005). The female louse lives for approximately 40 days and can lay over 100 eggs during her lifetime. Hatching time is approximately 7–10 days therefore if left untreated, individuals can become heavily infested.

Assessment

Clinical assessment of head, body and pubic lice includes:

- Presence of live adult lice
- Presence of immature lice
- Presence of nits and empty egg cases on hair shafts
- Presence of lice faeces or droppings on scalp and clothes
- Presence of excoriation, erythema, itch, scratching
- Signs of eczema, papules, vesicles, scaling, crusting
- Signs of infection, weeping exudate, swollen glands
- Previous infestations
- Family history/social history
- Previous treatments

Treatment of head, body and pubic lice

- Topical pediculicides
  - Malathion
  - Permethrin
  - Phenothrin
  - Carbaryl (unlicensed for crab lice)
- Physical combing for head lice
  - Using a fine toothed comb and hair conditioner
- Treatments involving alternative remedies such as tea-tree oil and other herbal substances

General advice

- Remain vigilant assess weekly
- Treat contacts and check close members of the family
- Launder bed linen at recommended temperature
- Avoid alcohol-based products if skin prone to eczema or excoriated
- Children can attend school once treatment strategy in place
- Avoid regular use or mixing and matching pediculicides treatments (encourages resistance).

Treatment with insecticides

Malathion is an organophosphate compound which inhibits the enzyme cholinesterase, in the louse. This means that the neurotransmitter substance, acetylcholine, accumulates resulting in interference of neurotransmission. Failure to transmit nerve impulses ultimately results in paralysis of the louse.

Carbaryl, also an organophosphate, kills lice in a manner similar to malathion.

The pyrethroids, permethrin and phenothrin, are synthetic compounds. They have a similar activity to the natural compound pyrethrum, which is extracted from plants of the Chrysanthemum family. These substances are rapidly absorbed across the louse cuticle and affect the sodium channels of the axons of louse neurones. The louse eventually dies following hyperexcitability, loss of coordination and prostration. These drugs however, do not always ensure destruction of lice ova.

Concerns regarding the use of insecticides

Aston *et al.* (1998) report that the three groups of chemicals currently used have had a good safety record over many years. The number of reported side effects recorded by the Adverse Drug Reactions section of the Committee on Safety of Medicines (CSM) is small. There have been only 26 reported side effects to malathion (in 18 individuals) during the past 25 years of use.

Carbaryl has recently had its legal status changed to a prescription-only medication (POM). It was found to cause tumour development in rats and mice that were exposed to high doses through their lifetime (Scowen 1995). The public responded to this information with some consternation, however it must be mentioned that carbaryl has been used for the past 40 years with no evidence of tumour development in humans. Children receive only a small dose, on a few occasions, whilst the laboratory animals received much higher doses, long term.

Topical application of malathion results in less absorption than with carbaryl (Maibach 1974). However, Sadler (1997) reports on current concerns regarding malathion. A pilot study indicates that following treatment with malathion, the amount of the drug excreted in the urine, is up to 10 times greater than in people with occupational exposure to the drug.

Management of head lice

There has been insufficient research and there is limited, quality scientific evidence on the treatment of head lice (Burgess 2000; National Prescribing Centre 1999; Aston *et al.* 1998). Head lice may be treated by mechanical clearance using the wet combing method; by using an insecticide preparation; or by other treatments involving alternative remedies such as tea-tree oil and other herbal substances. While there is some evidence that insecticides are effective, there is still no published evidence that mechanical methods such as 'Bug Busting' or alternative remedies are effective.

A diagnosis of head louse infection cannot be made with certainty unless a living, moving louse is found. Use of a louse comb is more efficient and much quicker than direct visual examination (Mumcuoglu *et al.* 2001) and according to Aston *et al.* (1998) the only reliable method of diagnosing current, active infection is by detection combing. The wet combing method is the best method of detecting live lice. This involves washing the hair in the normal manner, using an ordinary shampoo. An ordinary conditioner can then be applied to the hair. It is then combed with a fine tooth-detector comb whilst still wet. The hair should be combed in good lighting over a white cloth or paper towel in order to see the lice as they are removed. This process should take about15 minutes.

Treatment with insecticides

According to Aston *et al.* (1998) the cardinal rule before beginning treatment with insecticides, is that this treatment method should not be used unless a living, moving louse has been found on the head of at least one family member. Detection combing of all members should be undertaken, and only those found to be infected should be treated.

Malathion, carbaryl and the pyrethroids are all effective against head lice. In some health authorities, head lice are managed according to a local policy which rotates the use of these insecticides over a 2- or 3-year period. This attempts to reduce the risk of lice developing resistance to the preparations. These procedures of rotating insecticides are however, becoming less popular. Current

Contraindications

Malathion, carbaryl and the pyrethroids should not be applied to broken skin or secondarily infected skin. When used, care should be taken to avoid the eyes with all preparations.

Alcoholic lotions should be avoided in clients with asthma and in small children.

Permethrin should be avoided in pregnancy and if breastfeeding.

Side effects

Malathion, carbaryl and the pyrethroids may all cause skin irritation. In addition, permethrin may cause erythema, stinging, rashes and oedema.

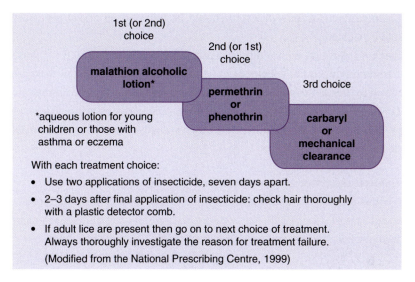

1st (or 2nd) choice

malathion alcoholic lotion*

2nd (or 1st) choice

permethrin or phenothrin

3rd choice

carbaryl or mechanical clearance

*aqueous lotion for young children or those with asthma or eczema

With each treatment choice:

- Use two applications of insecticide, seven days apart.
- 2–3 days after final application of insecticide: check hair thoroughly with a plastic detector comb.
- If adult lice are present then go on to next choice of treatment. Always thoroughly investigate the reason for treatment failure.

(Modified from the National Prescribing Centre, 1999)

Fig. 8.9 An example of a mosaic approach to the treatment of head lice.

UK practice involves individual management of each proven case using a mosaic of treatments (National Prescribing Centre, 1999). This is explained in Figure 8.9.

All three of these insecticidal groups are more effective as lotions rather than shampoos. In addition, the alcohol-based lotions are more effective than the aqueous lotions.

General points

Insecticides should not be used as prophylaxis for head lice. The wet combing method, however, may be used as a preventive measure. When prescribing a preparation, always observe the contraindications and precautions. Factors to consider are: age of the client, whether pregnant or breast feeding, the presence of other skin problems, and whether suffering from asthma.

Manufacturer's instructions must be followed for the specific preparation prescribed. A contact time of 12 hours is recommended for most lotions and liquids. The parent or client will need instruction on where and how it should be applied, and the length of time it must remain on the body to have its maximum effect.

A course of treatment for head lice is usually two applications of a preparation, 1 week apart. The second application aims to kill any remaining lice hatching from eggs that may have survived the first application.

Chlorine inactivates malathion, so clients should be advised to avoid swimming pools within 1 week of treatment.

Close contacts of those infested should be followed up and if necessary should be treated.

Further treatment with a different preparation will be required for those who remain symptomatic. Evidence of a secondary infection will necessitate a referral to the client's general practitioner for possible antibiotic therapy.

Li Wan Po (1990) suggests that in order to avoid excessive exposure to insecticides, gloves should be worn by those nurses involved in the application of these preparations.

Mechanical clearance

This whole method of treatment needs to be repeated every 3 to 4 days over a period of 2 weeks (Cook 1998). The presence of conditioner on the hair is thought to make the hair slippery and easier to detach the lice from the hair shaft.

Management of pubic lice

Malathion, phenothrin and permethrin will treat pubic lice effectively.

Contraindications and side effects

See previous section on the management of head lice. Alcoholic preparations are not recommended due to irritation of excoriated skin and genitalia. Aqueous preparations should be applied to all parts of the body and not just the axillae and groins.

Management of body lice

These lice only visit the skin for a supply of fresh blood, therefore clothes will be the main source of lice. All clothing and bedding of infested clients should be treated. After washing the clothes and bedding, use of a hot air tumble dryer will ensure destruction of lice and eggs remaining in the material. Insecticides may be necessary.

Scabies

Human scabies (see Figure 8.10) is a common parasitic infestation of the skin by the mite sarcoptes scabiei hominis. Occasional the animal scabies mite from a cat or dog can infest on human skin. The female mite burrows into the skin in order to lay eggs during reproduction. An acute itchy skin reaction can occur in response to mite faeces being present. Intense itch leads to scratching

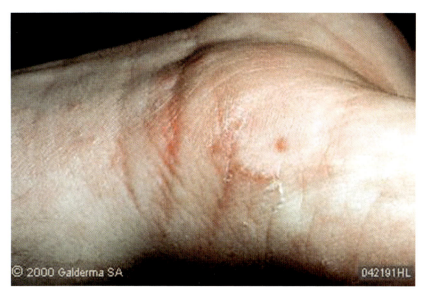

Fig. 8.10 Scabies (hand).

which results in an acute eczematous reaction around skin sites of infestation. Diffuse areas of eczema with vesicular papules can be widespread over the skin's surface. Excoriations, due to scratching, can become impetiginised due to secondary infection. Common sites for infestation are the lateral surfaces of fingers, interdigital webs of toes and fingers, palms of hands, wrists, penis and abdomen. The soles of the feet are commonly affected in babies and infants.

Visible linear burrows approximately 2–3 cm may be obvious which confirms diagnosis.

Transfer of the mite is by direct skin contact and scabies can spread very quickly within families. All relatives and partners in close contact with the affected person should be treated with an anti-scabies topical medication. Close contacts with no visible signs or symptoms of scabies should also be treated. Treatments should be undertaken at the time. A normal 60°C wash cycle will effectively treat any bed linen (BAD 2005).

Scabies is becoming increasingly common in the elderly population living in nursing homes or residential care homes. Vigilance on the part of health care workers is important in the assessment and successful management of scabies. Policies and protocols on prevention and management should be adhered in order to avoid widespread severe crusting infestation (Norwegian scabies) both for individuals and other residents.

Assessment

Assessment includes:

- onset, duration and distribution of rash
- type of lesions
- history of previous itchy skin and/or eczema
- family history of itchy skin
- evidence of linear burrows on affected skin
- previous treatments

Treatment

Scabies is always treated with topical application of anti-scabies medication (see lice).

- Malathion
- Permethrin
- Ivermectin (named patient basis for Norwegian scabies)
- Always treat all of the skin, including the scalp of children and soles of feet
- Treatment should be left on for 12 hours
- Retreat hands following washing
- Apply two treatments, 1 week apart (this treat hatching mites) (BAD 2005).

General skin care advice

- Gently wash and cleanse the skin with antimicrobial soothing emollients
- Avoid sharing wash cloths and towels
- Treat all family members and close contacts at same time
- Refrain from attending groups functions until skin treated and rash settled (e.g. nursery school)
- Launder bed linen at recommended temperature

Application of preparations

As alcoholic preparations are more likely to cause irritation to excoriated skin and the genitalia, aqueous preparations are preferable. They should be applied to clean, dry and cool skin, covering all body surfaces. A hot bath is not necessary and this may, indeed, increase systemic absorption and remove the drugs from their site of action. Particular attention should be paid to the finger webs and brushing lotion under the ends of the nails. The scalp, neck, face and ears do need to be treated in the very young and the elderly. These areas should also be treated in the immuno-compromised and those that are experiencing treatment failure.

Clients should not wash their hands after application, as hands need to be treated. Re-application is essential after handwashing.

All members of an affected household should be treated.

Apply two treatments, 1 week apart (this treat hatching mites).

Once only, normal laundering is sufficient for the client's clothing and bedding.

It is normal for itching to persist for 2 to 3 weeks after treatment, so itching should not be regarded as treatment failure. Calamine lotion or crotamiton cream may be applied to try and control itching. Itching that persists after 3 weeks may mean treatment failure and a referral to the general practitioner should be made to confirm the diagnosis.

When to refer

Scabies and lice are usually managed effectively in primary care as a home management and specialist referral is not advocated.

Consider referral if

- Skin condition fails to respond to recommended topical treatment
- Widespread secondary infection is apparent
- Evidence of Norwegian scabies (severe crusting scabies)
- Unsure of diagnosis

REFERENCES

Aston R, Duggal H & Simpson J (1998) *Head lice. Report for Consultants in Communicable Disease Control (CCDCs)*. The Public Health Medicine Environmental Group Executive Committee.

British Association of Dermatologists (2005) Patient Information Leaflets. London: BAD. www.bad.org.uk/public/leaflets/impetigo.asp (last accessed 5 May 2005).

British Association of Dermatologists (2005) Patient Information Leaflets. London: BAD. www.bad.org.uk/public/leaflets/erysipilas.asp (last accessed 5 May 2005).

British Association of Dermatologists (2005) Patient Information Leaflets. London: BAD. www.bad.org.uk/public/leaflets/molluscum.asp (last accessed 5 May 2005).

British Association of Dermatologists (2005) Patient Information Leaflets. London: BAD. www.bad.org.uk/public/leaflets/boils.asp (last accessed 5 May 2005).

British Association of Dermatologists (2005) Patient Information Leaflets. London: BAD. www.bad.org.uk/public/leaflets/herpessimplex.asp (last accessed 5 May 2005).

British Association of Dermatologists (2005) Patient Information Leaflets. London: BAD. www.bad.org.uk/public/leaflets/shingles.asp (last accessed 5 May 2005).

British Association of Dermatologists (2005) Patient Information Leaflets. London: BAD. www.bad.org.uk/public/leaflets/chronicparonichia.asp (last accessed 5 May 2005).

British Association of Dermatologists (2005) Patient Information Leaflets. London: BAD. www.bad.org.uk/public/leaflets/versicolor.asp (last accessed 5 May 2005).

British Association of Dermatologists (2005) Patient Information Leaflets. London: BAD. www.bad.org.uk/public/leaflets/lice.asp (last accessed 5 May 2005).

British Association of Dermatologists (2005) Patient Information Leaflets. London: BAD. www.bad.org.uk/public/leaflets/scabies.asp (last accessed 5 May 2005).

Burgess I. (2000) Head lice. *Clinical Evidence* 4: 975–8.

Clarke SC (2004) *Modern Medical Microbiology: The fundamentals.* London: Arnold. Chapter 54, pp. 170–2.

Galbraith A, Bullock S, Manias E, Hunt B & Richards A (1999) *Fundamentals of Pharmacology.* UK: Addison Wesley Longman Ltd.

Gillespie S & Bamford K (2000) *Medical Microbiology and Infection at a Glance.* Oxford: Blackwell Science Ltd. Chapter 50, pp. 106–7.

Gillespie S & Bamford K (2000) *Medical Microbiology and Infection at a Glance.* Oxford: Blackwell Science Ltd. Chapter 11, pp. 28–29.

Higgins EM, Fuller LC & Smith CH (2000) Guidelines for the management of *Tinea capitis. Br J Dermatol* 143: 53–8.

Lachapelle JM, Tennstedt & Marot L (1994) Atlas on Dermatology. Belgium: UCB Pharma Braine-l'Alleud.

Li Wan Po A (1990) Non-Prescription Drugs. 2nd edn. Oxford: Blackwell Scientific Publications.

Maibach HI (1974) Percutaneous penetration of some pesticides and herbicides in man. *Toxicol Appl Pharm* 28: 126–132.

Marks R (1983) *Practical Problems in Dermatology.* London: Martin Dunitz Ltd. Chapter 29, pp. 182–191.

Mumcuoglu KY, Friger M, Ioffe-Uspensky I, Ben-Ishaii F & Miller J (2001) Louse comb versus direct visual examination for the diagnosis of head louse infestations. *Pediat Dermatol* 18 (1): 9–12.

National Prescribing Centre (1999) Management of head louse infection. *Prescribing Nurse Bulletin* 1 (4): 13–16.

Sadler C (1997) A lousy headache. *Community Nurse* 3 (10): 8

Scowen P (1995) Government restricts the use of carbaryl for head lice. *Prof Care Mother and Child* 5 (6): 163–5.

Sterling JC, Handford-Jones S & Hudson PM (2001) Guidelines for the management of cutaneous warts. *Br J Dermatol* 144: 4–11.

Volk WA (1982) *Essentials of Medical Microbiology* (2nd Edn.). Philadelphia: JB Lippencott Co.

9

Skin cancer

Introduction

Managing patients with skin conditions in primary care will undoubtedly include skin cancer prevention. Prevention is an important aspect of the nurses role and involves three levels of intervention.

1. Education and self-care.
2. Screening for early disease with appropriate referral.
3. Specialist management and psychological intervention for patients with skin cancer.

This chapter aims to review skin cancer as a disease entity. Interventions which focus on health promotion through education and disease prevention strategies are highlighted.

Epidemiology of skin cancer

The incidence of skin cancer continues to rise within the white European adult population (Diepgen & Mahler 2002; De Gruijl 1999; WHO 1994). There are two main groups of skin cancer, melanoma skin cancer and non-melanoma skin cancer. Malignant melanoma is the least common but most lethal form of skin cancer with approximately 6000 new cases being diagnosed each year. Unfortunately the mortality rate for melanoma is high due to delayed diagnosis and intervention. Latest mortality figures indicate 2500 deaths per year from this disease (National Radiological Protection Board 2002; Office of National Statistics (ONS) 2000).

Non-melanoma skin cancers (basal cell carcinoma (BCC) and squamous cell carcinoma (SCC)) are more common with more than 46,000 new cases diagnosed each year. BCC rarely metastasise but can be disfiguring. SCC can metastasise and accounts for approximately 400 deaths per year in the UK (National Radiological Protection Board 2002).

Aetiology of skin cancer

Sunlight exposure is the most important contributing factor in the aetiology of all skin cancers (Bachman *et al.* 2001; Clyesdale *et al.* 2001; De-gruijl 1999; Leffel & Brash 1996; Godlee 1992; Brash *et al.* 1991):

- BCCs and SCCs arise in sun damaged skin.
- Precancerous skin lesions (Actinic Keratoses and Bowen's Disease) arise in sun damaged skin.
- BCCs and SCCs can also occur due to ionising radiation and burns to the skin.
- Polycyclic hydrocarbons (tars, mineral oils and soot), chemicals and viruses have been linked to the aetiology of SCCs.
- Melanoma is linked with frequent high-intensity sun exposure (sunburn) and childhood exposure. Other aetiological factors for melanoma include genetic disposition, skin type, family history, number of skin moles, environmental changes and sun seeking behaviour.

Acute intense short term UV sun damaged skin usually appears as erythema and blistering (sunburn). Long term chronic UV sun exposure ultimately leads to actinic skin damage, advanced ageing of the skin. This includes skin fragility, loss of dermal collagen and elastin, discolouration of the epidermis and development of deep set wrinkles. These changes are usually always seen on sun exposed sites of the hands, forearms, lower legs, face, neck and scalp. Precancerous lesions can arise in actinically damaged skin, the most common are Actinic Keratoses and Bowen's disease.

Common precancerous skin lesions

Actinic Keratoses (AK)

These lesions presents as hard, scaly dry lesions on the skin. They are usually numerous in number and frequently erthyema underlies the lesion. Actinic Keratoses have, if left untreated, a small percentage have the potential to progress to squamous cell carcinoma (National Radiological Protection Board (NRPB 2002)). These lesions can persist for many years become unsightly and cause loss of function especially those on the hands and fingers. Several treatment options are available for AKs and is dependent on number, site, age and general health of patient.

Bowen's Disease (BD)

Also known as intraepidermal carcinoma, Bowen's Disease presents as an erythematous scaly patch or plaque on the skin. These lesions will undergo neoplastic change to SCC if left untreated. Common sites are sun exposed areas of the skin such as the lower leg, arms, face and scalp.

Treatment for Actinic Keratoses and Bowen's Disease

Traditional managements include no treatment, or for larger lesions: excision surgery, curette and cautery, cryosurgery and topical chemotherapy creams. Increasing incidences in both an ageing population and a younger population has seen the development of non invasive treatment techniques. Newer treatment modalities include topical photodynamic therapy and topical immune response modulating creams. Daily moisturisation and sun-protection is integral to all management strategies for patients with sun damaged skin.

Malignant melanoma

Malignant melanoma (see Figure 9.1) is a tumour of the pigment producing cells of the skin (melanocytes). Melanocytes are dendritic cells of the skin which produce the pigment melanin in response to ultraviolet (UV) radiation. This is a natural protection mechanism against the carcinogenic effects of UV rays in solar radiation. Malignant melanoma appears on the skin as new or changing mole. Melanoma can occur anywhere on the skin and are commonly found on the legs of women and backs of men. Other sites include mucous membranes and the eye.

The most important diagnostic sign is history of CHANGE in mole characteristics. Change in size, shape or colour are early signs of malignant change. Itching, bleeding and crusting are more symptomatic and later changes (Mackie 2000).

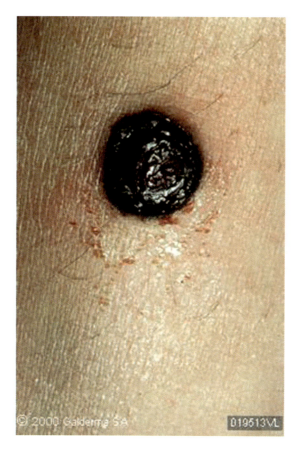

Fig. 9.1 Melanoma (ankle).

Key clinical features are described as the ABCD of melanoma:

A: Asymmetry (irregular shape).

B: Border (irregular, map like and prominences).

C: Colour (changes in colour or pigment to black, brown, blue and red).

D: Diameter (change in size or growth in diameter (>5 mm).

Types of melanoma

There are four main types of malignant melanoma (Mackie 1996):

- Superficial spreading malignant melanoma (SSMM)
  - Most common type
  - Initial lateral growth phase in epidermis prior to dermal invasion

- – ABCD of melanoma evident
- – Early recognition and treatment can facilitate cure.
- Nodular malignant melanoma
  - – Less common
  - – Appear as raised nodule on skin
  - – Frequently early dermal invasion
  - – Depth of dermal invasion predicts poorer prognosis.
- Lentigo maligna melanoma
  - – Typically sun-exposed sites (i.e. face, neck and hands)
  - – Arise from pre-existing benign lesion lentigo maligna (Hutchinson freckle)
  - – Appear as large flat pigmented lesion (>3 cm diameter)
  - – Vertical growth phase may occur after many years and indicates dermal invasion
  - – Early diagnosis and intervention can facilitate a cure.
- Acral lentigenous malignant melanoma
  - – Least common
  - – Arises on palms of hands and soles of feet
  - – Can appear as subungual lesions involving nail, nail bed and cuticle
  - – Delayed diagnosis carries poorer prognosis.

Treatment of malignant melanoma

Excision surgery is the first line management for all suspected primary cutaneous malignant melanoma (Mackie *et al.* 2001). This requires urgent referral (within 2 weeks) to a specialist trained in the surgical management of melanoma. Early diagnosis and surgical intervention can facilitate a cure for this potentially fatal form of skin cancer.

Secondary metastatic disease

The management of late stage malignant melanoma requires specialist medical, surgical and nursing intervention. Malignant melanoma will metastasis if not treated in the early stages of its development. Local, distant and widespread disseminated metastasis can occur. Treatment options include further surgery (excision secondary skin lesions, node dissection), bio-immuno-chemotherapy (interferon, interleukins, antibodies and cytotoxic agents) and radiotherapy (Mackie *et al.* 2001). At this stage the disease is highly aggressive with a fatal outcome. Treatment options at this stage are frequently experimental and palliative in nature.

Non-melanoma skin cancers (BCC, SCC)

Basal cell carcinoma

BCC (rodent ulcer – see Figure 9.2) is the most common form of skin cancer and appears on sun-exposed sites of the skin. BCCs are usually asymptomatic and rarely metastasise although they can spread and destroy local surrounding

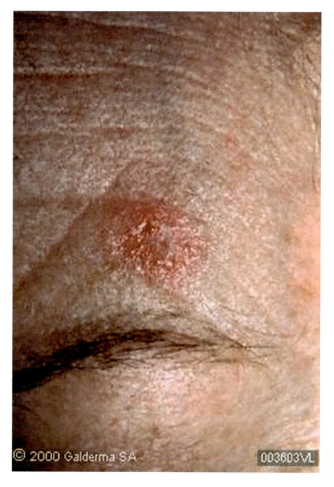

© 2000 Galderma SA   003603VL   **Fig. 9.2** Basal
cell carcinoma.

tissue. Frequently occur on face especially around the eye and lid, the scalp, the neck and behind the ear.

Clinical features

BCCs appear as:

- A red patch of skin which can be asymptomatic or itchy, painful or crusty.
- An open sore with central depression or ulcer which can bleed or crust but does not heal.
- Pale or white flat shiny scarred (atrophic) lesions.
- Red, pink or flesh coloured lesion with rolled pearly edge and central ulcer.
- Pink, red or flesh coloured lesion with visible telangectasia (minute vascular network) on border or edges.
- Firm smooth nodular lesions which are pink, red or flesh coloured.

Source: Mackie (1996).

Treatment of BCC

BCCs can be treated using invasive and non-invasive techniques.

Invasive techniques require specialist intervention and include:

- Simple excision
- Moh's surgery
- Curette and cautery (destructive surgical technique)
- Cryotherapy (destructive technique)
- Radiotherapy.

Non-invasive techniques can be facilitated in primary and secondary care, and include:

- Photodynamic therapy (PDT) (synergistic phototoxic effect of topical photosensitiser (methyl aminolevulinate), red light and oxygen.
- Topical application destructive creams (anti-metabolite fluorouracil, immuno-modulator imiquimod).

Source: Freak *et al.* (2000).

Squamous cell carcinoma

Like BCC, SCC (Figure 9.3) usually arises in sun-exposed sites such as the face, lips, ears and hands. It can also occur in scars, severely traumatised skin due

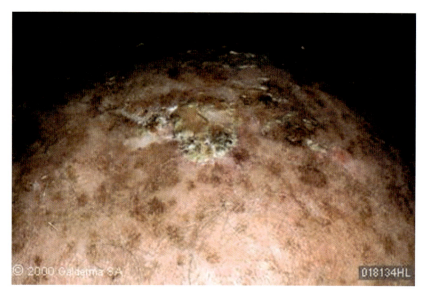

Fig. 9.3 Squamous cell carcinoma.

to burns, radiation and areas of chronic skin disease (venous ulcers and epidermolysis bullosa).

SCC is a slow growing lesion which is easily recognisable and treated. If left untreated, SCCs have the potential to metastasise to local and distant sites.

Clinical features

SCCs usually:

- Appear as non-healing indurated lesions
- Arise from pre-cancerous lesions (actinic keratoses and Bowen's disease)
- Are crusty scaly lesions which do not heal
- Are nodular lesions
- Are plaque like erythematous lesions
- Are verrucous lesions
- Ulcerated lesions.

Source: Freak *et al.* (2000) and Fleming (1995).

Treatment of SCC

Due to metastatic potential all suspected SCCs should be urgently referred to a specialist (within 2 weeks) (Department of Health 2001). Excision surgery is regarded as first line management. Other treatment options include Moh's surgery and radiotherapy.

Prevention of skin cancer

The key to skin cancer prevention is education (Buchanan 2001; Anti Cancer Council of Victoria 1999; Health Education Authority 1996; Koh 1996; Perkins 1993). Public education is essential if disease is to be prevented all together or recognised and treated at an early stage.

The nurse has a responsibility in health promotion and this can be utilised at three levels for skin cancer prevention.

Education and self-care

Public education needs to be implemented at a local level by health professionals, such as community nurses and pharmacists, to facilitate self-care. Education messages are included in the following:

- Avoid excessive sun exposure throughout life
- Protect children and babies from excessive sun exposure
- Enjoy the benefits of sunny weather without burning
- Avoid direct sunshine during mid-day hours
- Wear sun protective clothing, hats and sunglasses
- Apply high protection factor sunscreen (>SPF 15) prior to sun exposure
- Do not use sunscreens to prolong time out in the sun
- Protect skin everyday during hot spells and summer season, (at home, school, college and work) as well as when on holiday.

Source: Wessex Cancer Trust (2005), Cancer Research UK (2004) and Health Education Authority (1996).

Early screening

Early skin screening should begin in the home (Buchanan 2001). As health professionals we have responsibility to teach patients and clients how to scan and screen their own skin for any changing lesions, unhealing sores or abnormal moles. This strategy is aimed at reducing the time delay for patients seeking medical advice. This early screening strategy can then be backed up by screening in clinics, health centres and hospitals. Annual awareness days, weeks are frequently organised by health promotion teams, primary care and specialists to facilitate early diagnosis and educate the public.

Home screening guidelines are as follows:

- Review literature/leaflet which clearly shows clinical features of all skin cancers.
- Examine your skin every 6–12 months.
- Systematically *look and feel* for any changes in your skin, especially sun-exposed sites. Begin with scalp, face, neck, progress to arms, body and legs. Check hands, palms, soles of feet and nails.
- Ask a partner or family member to check 'difficult to see' areas (scalp and back) or alternatively use a mirror.
- Seek advice from your general practitioner (GP), pharmacist, primary care nurse if you are worried about any changing mole, unhealing sore, lesion or ulcer on your skin.

Source: Wessex Cancer Trust (2000).

Appropriate and timely referral for specialist intervention is within the remit of every primary care nurse. The referral pathway initially involves the GP who will then further assess the lesion and refer onto a specialist within recommendations of the Department of Health Cancer Plan (Department of Health 2001) as appropriate. This will be in line with NICE provisional recommendations for interventional procedures (NICE 2005).

Specialist intervention

Surgical intervention (excision surgery, Moh's surgery) is recognised as a first line management for BCCs (Telfer *et al.* 1999). This requires referral to the appropriate dermatologist or plastic surgeon in line with local guidelines and patient pathways. Cryotherapy, topical chemotherapy, curette and cautery and radiotherapy are also possible treatment options for BCCs. Pre-malignant lesions and primary non metastatic skin lesions can be treated with cryotherapy, curette and cautery and topical chemotherapy.

Recent developments in medicine and science have seen the introduction of non-invasive techniques for certain BCCs which have clear patients benefits, with regard to clinical efficacy, cost, access and cosmetic outcome. Some of the non-invasive techniques which are being undertaken are outlined below.

Non-invasive techniques: Photodynamic Therapy (PDT)

This is a simple and effective treatment for superficial BCCs, Bowen's Disease and actinic keratoses (Foley 2003; Horn *et al.* 2003; Szeimies *et al.* 2002; Solar *et al.* 2001).

Mode of action

PDT is a specific photochemical reaction within tumour cells due to the reaction of a photosensitising agent, red light and cellular oxygen. This reaction destroys targeted tumour cells by apotosis and necrosis. Topical PDT involves the preparation of the lesion by gentle descaling and removal of surface crusts. A photosensitising agent is then applied on and surrounding the lesion(s). Following protocol, the lesion is then illuminated with red light of an appropriate wavelength. This produces a photochemical reaction which results in target tumour destruction. A variety of agents and light sources have been used for topical PDT. Currently, for non melanoma skin tumours and precancerous lesions, the only photosensitising agent licensed in the UK is Methyl-Amino Levulinate.

Side effects

Side effects are usually transient and localised with reports of discomfort (e.g. stinging, burning and tingling sensations) being reported most commonly. A few patients report the discomfort as pain, and appears to be more common in skin-sensitive areas, such as the face, temples and scalp.

Post treatment, erythema is common with oedema, crusting and scabbing. Topical anti-inflammatory corticosteroid may be applied once or twice daily to relieve the erythematous response. Very rarely erosion or ulceration has been reported. Healing is usually uncomplicated with minimal or no scarring.

Clinical follow-up is usually at 3 months to ensure complete resolution of the tumour.

Topical agents

Topical Fluorouracil 5%

Mode of action

Topical Fluorouracil 5% is a prescription-only medication for BCCs and pre-cancerous skin lesions. It is classified as an anti-metabolite. Antimetabolite preparations are similar in structure to the natural metabolites that are required for growth and division of rapidly growing neoplastic and normal cells. Antimetabolites prevent normal cellular function by replacing natural metabolites. Fluorouracil is applied carefully and specifically to the lesion(s) in a thin layer once or twice daily. The BCCs should then be covered with a light dressing. Although local variations in management regimens may differ, the average length of treatment time is 3–4 weeks.

Side effects

Local intense irritation and inflammation is likely; therefore, small areas of skin should be treated at least one time (maximum 500 cm^2). Contact with eyes and mucous membranes should be avoided.

Imiquimod

Mode of action

Imiquimod is a topical immunomodulator licensed for the treatment of basal cell carcinoma and actinic keratoses. Immunomodulating agents are preparations that modify the body's immune responsiveness. Immunomodulators affect the function of leucocytes, and alter the level of cytokines (i.e. the secretions produced by leucocytes) and immunoglobulins. Imiquimod should be applied thinly five times a week for six weeks at night.

Side effects

Application to normal skin, inflamed skin and open wounds should be avoided. Local reactions include itching, pain and erythema (BNF 2005).

Diclofenac sodium

Mode of action

Diclofenac sodium is a non-steroidal anti-inflammatory drug (NSAID). The NSAIDs act by suppressing the formation of prostaglandin. Prostaglandins are fatty acids which act as chemical messengers released to co-ordinate local

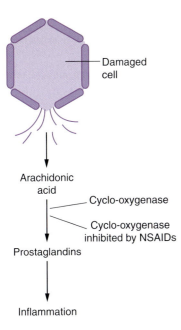

Arachidonic
acid

Cyclo-oxygenase

Cyclo-oxygenase
inhibited by NSAIDs

Prostaglandins

Inflammation

Fig. 9.4 The action of aspirin and other NSAIDs.

cellular activity. These substances, formed by most cells of the body, and released in response to a number of stimuli, are major contributors to inflammation and pain. NSAIDs act by blocking the enzyme cyclo-oxygenase, responsible for converting arachidonic acid (a fatty acid released from cell membranes following injury), into prostaglandin (see Figure 9.4). The analgesic action of these preparations are therefore largely local, peripherally acting in damaged tissue, rather than centrally in the brain.

Diclofenac sodium is a topical agent licensed for the treatment of precancerous skin lesions. It should be applied thinly two times daily for 60–90 days.

Caution

Apply with gentle massage only. Contact with eyes, mucous membranes and inflamed or broken skin should be avoided. Preparation should be discontinued if a rash develops. Large amounts applied topically may result in systemic effects including hypersensitivity and asthma (BNF 2005).

REFERENCES

Anti Cancer Council of Victoria (1999) *Sun Smart Evaluation Studies 1996/7–1997/8 Cancer Control Program*. Related Research Evaluation Number 6. Anti-Cancer Council of Victoria. Australia: Carlton.

Bachman F, Buechner SA, Wernli M, Strebel S & Erb P (2001) Ultraviolet light down regulates CD95 ligand and trail receptors facilitating keratosis and squamous cell carcinoma formation. *J Invest Dermatol* 117: 59–66.

Bastuji-Garin S & Diepgen TL (2002) Cutaneous melanoma, sun exposure and sunscreen use: epidemiological evidence. *Br J Dermatol Suppl* 146 (61): 24–30.

BNF (2005) British Medical Association (BMA). Royal Pharmaceutical Society of Great Britain (RPSGB). London: BMA and RPSGB.

Brash D, Rudolf J, Simon JA, Lin A, McKenna GL, Baden HP, Halperin AJ & Ponten J (1991) A role for sunlight in skin cancer: UV-induced p53 mutations in squamous cell carcinoma. *Professional National Academic Scientific USA* 88: 10124–8.

Buchanan P (2001) Skin cancer. *Nurs Stand* 15 (45): 45–52.

Clyesdale GJ, Dandie GW & Konrad-Muller H (2001) Ultraviolet light induced injury: immunologicical and inflammatory effects. *Immunol Cell Biol* 79: 547–68.

Cancer Research UK (2004) Sun Smart Campaign. London: CRUK.

De-Gruijl FR (1999) Skin cancer and solar radiation. *Eur J Cancer* 35 (14): 2003–9.

Department of Health (2001) The NHS Cancer plan: a plan for investment, a plan for reform. London: HMSO.

Diepgen TL & Mahler V (2002) The epidemiology of skin cancer. *Br J Dermatol Suppl* 146 (61): 1–6.

Freak J, Buchanan P, Sullivan A, Wheelhouse C & Warne J (2000) *The Prevention and Management of Skin Cancer: Open Learning Workbook*. Bournemouth University.

Foley P (2003) Clinical efficacy of methyl aminolevulinate (metvix) photodynamic therapy. *J Dermatol Treatment* 14 (Suppl 3): 15–22.

Godlee F (1992) Dangers of ozone depletion. In: *Health and the Environment* (Eds Godlee F & Walker A). BMJ: London.

Haller JC, Cairnduff F, Slack G *et al.* (2000) Routine double treatments of superficial basal cell carcinomas using aminolevulinic acid based photodynamic therapy. *Br J Dermaotol* 143: 1270–4.

Health Education Authority (1996) *Sun Know How Campaign*. London: HEA.

Horn M, Wolf P, Wulf HC *et al.* (2003) Topical methyl aminolevulinate photodynamic therapy in patients with basal cell carcinoma prone to complications and poor cosmetic outcome with conventional treatment. *Br J dermatol* 149: 1242–9.

Koh H (1996) Prevention and early detection strategies for melanoma and skin cancer. *Arch Dermatol* 132: 436–43.

Leffell DJ & Brash DE (1996) Sunlight and skin cancer. *Scient Am* 275 (1): 38–43.

Mackie R (2000) *Primary Cutaneous Malignant Melanoma: A Guide to Clinical Diagnosis, Differential Diagnosis and Current Treatment*. Edinburgh: Lothian Print.

Mackie R (1996) *Skin Cancer: An Illustrated Guide to the Aaetiology, Clinical Features, Pathology and Management of Benign and Malignant Cutaneous Tumours*. London: Dunitz.

Mackie R, Murray D, Rosin RD, Hancock B & Miles A (Eds) (2001) *The Effective Management of Cutaneous Malignant Melanoma*. London: Aesculapius Press.

NRPB (2002) *Health effects from Ultraviolet Radiation; Documents of the NRPB*. Didcot, National Radiological Protection Board 13(1) Chapter 7; pp. 125–90.

Office of National Statistics (2000) Cancer survival in England and wales 1991 Health Statistics Quarterly 6: 71–80.

Perkins P (1993) Prevention through education. Child Health 1 (3): 111–21.

Solar AM, Warloe T, Berner A & Giercksky KE (2001) A follow up study of recurrence and comesis in completely responding superficial and nodular basal cell carcinomas treated with methyl-5-aminolaevulinate-based photodynamic therapy alone and with prior curettage. *Br J Dermatol* 145: 467–71.

Szeimies RM, Karrer S, Radakovic-Fijan S, Tanew A, Calzavara-Pinton PG, Zane C, Sideroff A, Hempel M, Ulrich J, Proebstle T, Meffert H *et al.* (2002) *J Am Acad Dermatol* 47 (2): 258–62.

Telfer NR, Colver GB & Bowers PW (1999) Guidelines for the management of Basal Cell carcinoma. *Br J Dermatol* 141: 415–23.

World Health Organisation (1994) Environmental Health Criteria 160; ultraviolet radiation. Geneva: WHO.

Wessex Cancer Trust (2005) www.wessexcancer.org (last accessed 20 April 2005).

Wessex Cancer Trust (2000) *Marc's Line Self-examination Leaflet*. WCT Southampton.

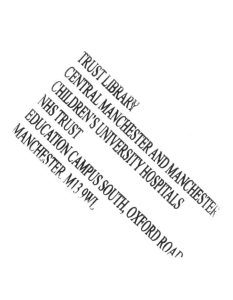

Index